Young people living
with cancer

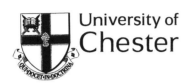

University of
Chester

Young people living with cancer

Implications for policy and practice

Anne Grinyer

Open University Press

Open University Press
McGraw-Hill Education
McGraw-Hill House
Shoppenhangers Road
Maidenhead
Berkshire
England
SL6 2QL

email: enquiries@openup.co.uk
world wide web: www.openup.co.uk

and Two Penn Plaza, New York, NY 10121–2289, USA

First published 2007

A catalogue record of this book is available from the British Library

ISBN-10: 0 335 22154 8 (pb) 0 335 22155 6 (hb)
ISBN-13: 978 0 335 22154 7 (pb) 978 0 335 22155 4 (hb)

Library of Congress Cataloguing-in-Publication Data
CIP data applied for

Typeset by YHT Ltd, London
Printed by Printed in Poland by OZ Graf. S. A.
www.polskabook.pl

The *McGraw-Hill* Companies

This book is dedicated to the memory of George whose life, illness and death have touched the lives of so many people, and to his parents Helen and Geoff. It is also for all the young people who shared part of their journey with me.

Now is not a good time.

(Steven, diagnosed at 18 with Hodgkin's disease)

Contents

Participants

The following details are for easy reference for readers. Further information on how each participant was recruited is included in Appendix I, Methods.

Young adults and those with them at the interview

Adrian (and his partner Cindy's mother)
A scaffolder diagnosed at 18 with testicular cancer, living with girlfriend Cindy and her parents.

Aidan (and his mother)
At school when diagnosed at 15 with osteosarcoma in his pelvis.

Charlotte (and her grandmother)
At college when diagnosed at 17 with a liver tumour.

Craig
Diagnosed at 18 with testicular cancer.

Dawn
A hairdresser diagnosed at 20 with acute lymphoblastic leukaemia.

Devika
At school when diagnosed with acute lymphoblastic leukaemia.

Donovan
At college doing a joinery course when diagnosed with osteosarcoma at 17.

Emma (and her partner Gary and children Brooklyn and Chloe)
A full-time mother when diagnosed at 21 with Hodgkin's lymphoma.

Gemma
A nurse on an orthopaedic ward, 23 when diagnosed with Hodgkin's lymphoma.

Hoody (and his mother and father)
At school when diagnosed with osteosarcoma at the age of 16.

James
At school when diagnosed with acute lymphoblastic leukaemia at 16.

Kelly (and her baby daughter)
A wife and mother of a baby when diagnosed at 26 with lymphoma.

Lucy (and her mother)
At school when diagnosed at 13 with lymphoma.

Luke (and his aunt)
At school when diagnosed at 16 with Ewing's sarcoma in his hip.

Marc
An apprentice in a factory and at college when diagnosed at 20 with testicular cancer.

Mark
A butcher already married when diagnosed with testicular cancer at 21 who has since fathered two daughters naturally.

Michelle (and her mother)
Newly graduated from university when diagnosed with an adrenal tumour at 21.

Nathan
An apprentice joiner and at college when diagnosed at 17 with Hodgkin's disease.

Nicola
A play worker with infants and pregnant when diagnosed at 19 with an ovarian tumour, has since had a baby naturally.

Philip
A trainee Outward Bound instructor when diagnosed at 20 with bowel cancer.

Ricky (and his mother)
At school when diagnosed with leukaemia at the age of 15.

Ross (and his partner Hannah)
A self-employed agricultural/haulage contractor when diagnosed with osteosarcoma at 23.

Ruth
At school when diagnosed at 14 with anaplastic large cell lymphoma, extract taken from her previously written account.

Steve
A student in his early twenties, a long-term survivor of childhood cancer diagnosed when he was 10.

Steven
A heavy goods vehicle apprentice when diagnosed at 18 with Hodgkin's disease.

Thomas
At school when diagnosed with osteosarcoma in his knee.

Toni (and her mother)
About to go to university when diagnosed at 19 with lymphoma.

Vicky (and her mother)
At school when diagnosed at 15 with leukaemia.

Health care and other professionals interviewed

Alison: Lead cancer nurse in a non-specialist setting.

Cat: Activity coordinator on the specialist ward.

Deborah: Staff nurse on the specialist ward.

Diane: Sister on the specialist ward.

Hazel: Medical social worker in a non-specialist setting

Dr James: General practitioner at a university practice.

Simon: Learning mentor on the specialist ward.

Sue: Lead Macmillan clinical nurse specialist for teenagers and young adults.

Other sources

Sunita's sister who agreed to talk about her sister's illness for the research, but not to be recorded.

In addition, informal discussions were held with a number of health professionals and support staff. The information they offered, while not attributed, has offered an additional perspective and has contributed to my understanding of the context of care.

Foreword

My research on young adults and cancer was inspired by the life, illness and death of George. George was a student of 23 when he died in 1999 after a four-year battle with osteosarcoma. Throughout the duration of George's illness and treatment, his parents, Helen and Geoff, faced immense difficulties, many of which they believed stemmed from his age and life stage. These challenges exacerbated the predictable distress of caring for a son or daughter with a life-threatening illness, but a search for information on how to manage the situation proved fruitless as it appeared little or no research had been published on the psychological and social impact of cancer in this age group.

After George's death, Helen and Geoff set up a memorial trust to fund research, focusing on the impact on the parents of young adults with cancer, and this resulted in the kind of publications they believed would have assisted them in their struggle to support George (Grinyer 2002a, 2002b, 2004a, 2005, 2006a, 2006b, in press; Grinyer and Thomas 2001, 2004). The first phase of the research provided an understanding of the effect on parents and families supporting their sons and daughters through the cancer journey. However, after the completion of this phase of the research, there was a strong feeling from all concerned that the voices of the young people should also be heard. This volume is the result of listening to their stories and is based on the narratives of teenagers and young adults with cancer; the issues raised are those that were of significance to them.

The research began soon after the NICE (National Institute for Health and Clinical Excellence) Guidance (NICE 2005a) for children and young people with cancer was published and responds to its concerns about the provision of age-appropriate care. The hope is that the young adults' first-hand accounts will contribute to understanding the needs of the age group in relationship to their life stage and consequently the implications for care will be clarified. One of the aims has been to appreciate what it means to be a young adult with cancer – to identify the essence of the experience from the perspective of the young people. If families, professionals and policy-makers can understand better the impact on the lives of the young adults, it will be more likely that both formal and informal support services will be able offer age-appropriate care based on needs identified by the young adults themselves.

Many aspects of the research have proved challenging, this is a hard to reach group and the barriers to accessing them have at times appeared almost insurmountable.[1] However, after much encouragement, support and the sterling work of key health care professionals, the research has resulted in this volume.

Anne Grinyer

Note

1   Details of the difficulties of access are recounted in the discussion of the methodology in Appendix I.

Acknowledgements

This book could not have been written without the support and practical help of many people. The research was made possible by the George Easton Memorial Trust and those who support it financially, to whom I am very grateful. My thanks also go to all the healthcare professionals who trusted me to speak to their patients, to Clare and Jose for their sterling work in recruiting participants, and to Sue Morgan for her continuous support over several years. I am indebted to Geoff, Judith, Jane, Julie and David for their helpful comments on early drafts of this volume, to Anthony for his much-needed technical help and to Helen who as always acted as my guide, proof reader and unofficial research assistant. However, my biggest thanks go to all the young people with cancer who agreed to talk to me; they gave me their time and shared their experiences with generosity. This book is a tribute to their courage.

1   Setting the scene

Thankfully, cancer is uncommon in young adulthood, as Birch et al. (2003) document, numbers are low and accounted for only 0.5 per cent of all cancers in 1999 but this figure had risen to 0.6 per cent in 2000 (Birch 2005). Nevertheless, despite its relative rarity, cancer is the most common natural cause of death among teenagers and young adults and is exceeded in incidence only by accidental death (Albritton and Bleyer 2003; Birch et al. 2003).

Birch et al. (2003: 2622) report the UK national incidence rates in young people: those aged 12–14 at 10.1, aged 15–19 at 14.4 and aged 20–24 at 22.6 per 100,000 population and according to Albritton and Bleyer (2003) in 15–19-year-olds, cancer occurs at nearly twice the rate observed in 5–14-year-olds. Thus we can see that the incidence of cancer rises during the teenage years and into young adulthood.

Furthermore, there seems to have been a significant increase in young adult cancers over the past 20–30 years. Examining temporal trends in incidence from 1979–2000 in England, Birch (2005: 22) shows that while there are differences in the increase of specific cancers, the overall increase during this period has climbed from 15.41 to 19.80 per 100,000, a rise of approximately 30 per cent. Selby et al. (2005: 271) report the increase from 1975–2000 as rising from 16 per 100,000 a year to 24 per 100,000 a year – an increase of 45 per cent over the period. Thomas et al. (2006: 303) use figures from the Australian Institute of Health and Welfare that show a marked rise. Between 1983 and 2001, the incidence of cancer in 15–30-year-olds in Australia rose by over 30 per cent for reasons that Thomas et al. acknowledge are not clear.

The Teenage Cancer Trust reports that:

> In the last 30 years the incidence of cancer in the teenage and young adult group has increased by 50% and for the first time ever, the number of teens with cancer now exceeds the number of children with cancer ... Teenagers contract some of the most aggressive cancers that are made worse by their growth spurts.
>
> (Teenage Cancer Trust Health Facts website 2006a)

The rise in incidence for adolescents can be contrasted with a comparatively lower increase for children. The findings of Steliarova-Foucher et al. (2004), researchers who have tracked the incidence of cancer across Europe since the 1970s, show that over three decades the overall incidence has increased each year by 1 per cent in children but by 1.5 per cent in adolescents. Using data from the USA, Decker et al. (2004) report a 30 per cent rise in the past 20 years for adolescents, compared to a 10 per cent increase for younger children.

There is, however, an additional concern. According to Thomas et al. (2006), improvements in outcomes for young adults lag well behind the advances achieved for children and older adults; the improvement in survival of young people between 1973–2001 being half that seen in children or older adults. These findings are endorsed by Albritton and Bleyer (2003) who say that the improvement in the survival rate among adolescents in the USA has been 50 per cent less than for children and older adults. However, despite these comparatively worse outcomes, there is evidence of a decline in mortality. Based on a study of selected cancers among 15–24-year-olds from 1965–98 in Europe, the USA and Japan, Levi et al. (2003: 2611) document a decrease in mortality of 40 per cent. Nevertheless, the decline in mortality from leukaemias and other neoplasms was smaller between the ages of 15–24 than it was for children. What improvements there have been are attributed largely to better treatments and inclusion in multi-centre clinical trials.

Haase and Phillips (2004: 145) attribute the relatively poorer outcomes to: unique biologies of cancer, unique medical and psychosocial needs, under-representation in clinical trials, and facing physical, emotional and social challenges that are experienced as particularly difficult. Yet these authors suggest that young adults with cancer can be rendered 'invisible' as research data frequently do not distinguish the age group clearly from that of children or older adults, and in addition they 'rarely receive care in settings designed to meet their unique needs' (2004: 145–6). So we can see that there is a need to develop services targeted at teenage and young adult cancer patients. According to Albritton and Bleyer:

> Adolescents with cancer must be recognised as a subgroup of oncology patents with specific needs requiring dedicated interest and management ... A further consideration is that the physical, emotional and social challenges posed by cancer in adolescent and early adult life are often unique and especially difficult for patients, families and health care providers alike; these needs remain largely unstudied and unmet.
>
> (2003: 2854)

Birch et al. (2003) suggest that provision of these unmet needs should be based on high quality statistics. However, while statistical data are central to establishing the aetiology of disease, and to the provision of appropriate medical care, an additional level of insight is needed. If, as Albritton and

Bleyer (2003: 2595) argue, adolescents have many of the factors associated with 'non-adherence', an in-depth understanding of the characteristics of teenagers and young adults and their experience of the illness and treatments must also play an integral part in designing services. This book attempts to fill the 'unstudied' gap through a qualitative approach that provides knowledge on what it is like to be a young adult with cancer. It is to be hoped that such an understanding will contribute to the provision of optimal care not only medically, but also help to support the cancer journey socially, emotionally and psychologically.

The provision of adolescent services

A press release from the Teenage Cancer Trust (TCT) issued early in 2004 was entitled 'Teenagers miss out on cancer care' and warned that adolescents were 'falling through the gap' of child and adolescent services while every day in the UK six 15–24-year-olds are diagnosed with cancer. Since that press release was issued, there has been a growing recognition that specialist services are required to address the physical, social and emotional needs of a group that has not been well served. One of the responses to this need was the National Institute for Health and Clinical Excellence (NICE 2005a) Guidance for children and young people with cancer. A press release issued by NICE (2005b) contains the following quote from Peter Littlejohns, Executive Lead for the guidance:

> The distinct needs of young people with cancer have been increasingly recognised over recent years. Many young people do not feel comfortable within the paediatric setting, but they have unique needs that may not be addressed within adult services. This guidance identifies the specific age-related services that need to be provided to ensure that children and young people with cancer receive the best care, and their families the support they need, no matter where they live in England and Wales.
>
> (NICE 2005b: 1)

There is a clear recognition in this statement that adolescence and young adulthood is a time of life that brings with it special requirements in terms of appropriate medical services. Jeremy Whelan, a consultant oncologist specializing in teenage cancer, who also chairs the TYAC (Teenagers and Young Adults with Cancer) Board, says that while there are 'shortfalls in care and inequalities of access to special expertise' (2005: 12), the UK's recognition of teenagers and young adults as a distinct group is unparalleled anywhere in the world. Making reference to the NICE Guidance (2005a), he says that there are signs of real commitment from government to support the necessary provision of services for a group that falls between children's and adult services. The key issues are, according to Whelan: 'Poor disease outcomes and low inclusion in clinical trials ... [and] how to support young people living away from major centres where inevitably specialist cancer treatment services must be concentrated' (2005: 12).

Interestingly, the UK is not the only country to be addressing the needs of this particular age group: in Australia, Dr David Thomas of the Peter Mac-Callum Cancer Centre in Melbourne has stated that for young people in this 'grey zone' treatment was dispersed through many centres that did not provide the 'specialised infrastructure needed for the dedicated psychosocial support ... and appropriate environment of peer support' (2006). Thomas identifies a number of age-related characteristics that contribute to the difficulty of providing appropriate care: balancing young people's need for autonomy and independence with the demands of their parents, managing the effect of cancer on intimacy and sexuality, ensuring that education continues despite the illness and treatment, facilitating social development and ensuring that young cancer patients do not become isolated from their social support network.

Tim Eden, the UK's first professor of Teenage and Adolescent Cancer (HERO 2005), identifies key questions that need to be answered if specialist services are to deliver care that translates into increased survival rates:

- Who does develop cancer in the age range 13–24 years?
- What is the tumour profile and causation?
- What is survival rate?
- Is referral late and inappropriate?
- Who treats these patients?
- Why is trial entry so low?
- Why is there such a divide between adult and child services?
- What special support is required?

(Eden 2006)

It is beyond the scope of this volume to attempt to answer all these questions. However, if the cancer journey can be understood better through young adults' own accounts, the provision of appropriate care and services may contribute to the improvement of outcomes.

One of the challenges to the appropriate provision of care is the difficulty in locating a group that occupies what Thomas (2006) refers to as the 'grey zone'. This raises the question of whether the group is paediatric, adult or something distinct in itself – and if this group is a distinct entity, what are its defining characteristics. This is a question that this volume attempts to answer.

The development of the NICE Guidance for children and young people with cancer (2005a) signifies recognition that the age group requires the provision of services that is age-appropriate. There is an acknowledgement in the NICE Guidance that the original title of the document was to have been 'Child and Adolescent Cancer' but it became clear that an arbitrary upper age limit was unacceptable. In the document there is recognition that children's and adult services may be experienced as inappropriate by young people of 19 and older who are too old for children's services yet too young for the adult services catering for a predominantly elderly population and that they should have unhindered access to age-appropriate support and facilities. It seems that the title of 'children and young people', while not setting an upper age limit, suggests that the range of life stages represented in this spectrum can be considered together satisfactorily. However, the document addresses the problematic definitions of childhood and adulthood as follows:

> There are various definitions of the boundary between childhood and adulthood used by society, some of which define a legal entitlement or access to services ... Children are as different from each other as they are from adults. The guidance is based around three main groups – children, teenagers and young adults – although the term 'young people' is used throughout when it is unnecessary to differentiate between teenagers and young adults.
>
> (NICE 2005a: 12)

This quote captures one of the challenges for the provision of care for this age group, as there are not only a wide range of life stages within the category, but unpredictable and variable rates of maturity, need and family relationships. Adolescence is a period of transition between childhood and adulthood – a kind of 'no man's land' – when neither childhood nor adult services are experienced as appropriate (Apter 2001; Brannen et al. 1994; Grinyer 2002a). It encompasses young people around whom it is difficult to draw impermeable age-related boundaries, but who nevertheless have certain age-specific needs. For example, there are great differences even within a group of those aged 16–18. Some will have left school, be in full-time jobs and may be parents, while others will be dependent on parents, still in full-time education and only beginning to leave childhood. There will be gender differences and even differences from one day to the next when a fiercely independent teenager reverts to almost infantile dependency if feeling frightened or insecure; and what is more likely to cause such an ontological crisis than the diagnosis of a life-threatening illness? As George and Hutton (2003: 2663) claim, they may 'oscillate between extreme independence and crass juvenility'. The transitional life stage of young adulthood is by its very nature not a linear process that moves smoothly or predictably from dependence to independence, but rather a fluctuating trend that can be unpredictable and exacerbated by life-threatening illness.

During this transitional period, relationships with parents are changing, independence is being sought, careers are being established and new relationships are being formed outside the family and with sexual partners. As part of this process of separation, the onus for health-related decisions that were once the preserve of the parents (usually the mother), becomes increasingly that of the young adult (Grinyer 2002a). Additionally, this age group is known for its risk-taking behaviour as the young adults test the boundaries imposed by authority figures such as parents and professionals. According to Craig (2006: 109), part of this process is to challenge previously accepted family beliefs and to identify more intensively with a peer group. These life-stage issues create a complex context which may be coupled with the young adults' lack of awareness of the implications of symptoms and/or an unwillingness to seek medical advice; and even when they do present symptoms, their understanding may be incomplete or flawed (Albritton and Bleyer 2003: 2595). When combined with the limitations of speedy and appropriate diagnoses (Whiteson 2005) and the ability to provide appropriate services, we can see that the age group presents a particular challenge for health professionals attempting to optimize outcomes.

This combination of factors may result in life-threatening illness remaining unrecognized and untreated. Even when a diagnosis is made, the setting of care may, as the NICE press release (2005b) suggests, fall between services which are experienced as inappropriate. Thus the transitional stage of young adulthood carries with it implications for the success of cancer treatment and the consequent survival rates.[1] The life experiences for this age range of 'children and young adults' may be more disparate than at almost any other age, making the development of policy to meet the needs of the age group a challenging task. Nevertheless, the NICE Guidance (2005a) attempts to incorporate a consideration of the particular issues that pertain to older teenagers and young adults in its policy document. Included among the key recommendations for the provision of care are the following:

- There is a clear organizational structure for the services.
- All aspects of care should be undertaken by appropriately trained staff.
- Principal treatment centres are identified for cancer types with associated referral pathways.
- Shared care arrangements are established that identify a lead clinician.
- Appropriately skilled key workers should be identified to support the patients and their families by coordinating their care across the system, providing information and assessing and meeting their needs for support.

- All care for children and young people under 19 years old must be provided in age-appropriate facilities.
- All treatment sites should be subject to peer review.
- National guidance is followed.

(NICE 2005a: 7–8)

If such policies are to be put into practice, there needs to be a clear understanding of what the (changing and changeable) needs of the age group are, and that a 'one size fits all' approach would be a relatively meaningless and problematic basis for policy. However, despite the clear differences between the life experiences of the young people, it is nevertheless a fundamental principle of this research that those in the age group have more that unites them than divides them. Whatever point they occupy on the continuum, they are all on the threshold of life with hopes and aspirations for a future of as yet unfulfilled plans and ambitions, and at a vulnerable time in their lives when their sense of identity may be fragile (Grinyer 2002a).

Discussions with key staff delivering care in specialist facilities suggest that they have a clear idea of what their patients need and value but much of their 'evidence' is based on informal observation rather than any systematic research. In a culture of evidence-based medicine, it is necessary to document how the provision of services is perceived and experienced by the young people themselves through examining the range of needs and emotions and the fluidity of states that are characteristic of this life stage.

The research, its participants and the structure of the book

While an insight into their experience was provided by parents (Grinyer 2002a), it is necessary to enter the life world of the young people with cancer in an attempt to understand the experience from their own perspective and through their stories.

The age group from which the sample is drawn has been somewhat arbitrarily defined as 16–25, yet the boundaries are hard to draw with precision. While the original data that form the basis for this volume were collected from young people between the ages of 16–26, some of them had been diagnosed at an earlier age and could therefore reflect on what it is like to be a 14-year-old with cancer. Their changing and changeable needs are addressed through an analysis of the fieldwork in an attempt to show that the concept of age-appropriate care needs to be understood in relationship to where on the continuum the young person is, chronologically, socially and emotionally. Indeed, the use of the term 'age-appropriate care' is only meaningful if it is not used as a mantra to cover a range of different needs.

The following six chapters are based on original data derived from interviews with young people with cancer. The chapters have each been organized around a central theme, though it has been difficult to draw boundaries around many of the issues which are interconnected and overlapping. Nevertheless, the thematic nature of the discussion is designed so that health professionals involved in the care of the young people, policy-makers who plan the provision of care and young people who experience care, can access issues of interest and concern to them with ease.

The empirical chapters begin by examining barriers to diagnosis and this is followed by a chapter that focuses on the effect of the setting of care. The remaining interview-based chapters address more personal themes: the loss of independence and normality, the disruption to life trajectory, the impact on friendships and social activities, how changes to physical appearance are experienced and, finally, the effect of the illness and its treatment on sexuality and fertility. The final chapter considers how the material presented thus far can inform policy and practice.

There are many quotes from the young adults contained in the text, and this is primarily because the verbatim words of the participants speak more powerfully than any summary or synopsis that I provide. I tell their stories in an albeit fragmented way, but nevertheless attempt to give the young people voice to communicate what it is like to have the course of their lives transformed by a cancer diagnosis.[2]

Notes

1   The effect of the transitional life stage has been explored in relationship to life-threatening illness and the impact on the family in Grinyer (2002a) from the parents' perspective. The introductory chapter of that volume could equally as well introduce this one. Because it may be useful for readers to have access to literature and theories relating to the particular age group, relevant extracts are reproduced in Appendix II on p. 164.

2   Throughout the process of collecting the data from the young adults with cancer I was mindful of the ethical issues and the sensitivity required in my interactions with them. For those readers who are interested in how the data were gathered and the consent procedures involved, there is a full discussion of the methods and ethical considerations in Appendix I on p. 154.

2   Diagnosis

The swift diagnosis of cancer in young adults has been identified as a key factor in their survival. According to the NICE Guidance (2005a), a GP will on average see a child under 15 with cancer only once every 20 years. The figure for the over-15s is not specified, nevertheless, the incidence in the 15–24-year age range is also likely to be small and GPs are thus unlikely to encounter many in their practice. The non-specific nature of many of the symptoms, coupled with the multiplicity of cancer types, may combine with a lack of experience and result in a GP not suspecting a cancer diagnosis in this age group, thus contributing to late diagnosis. The NICE Guidance states that some deaths among young people occur before a cancer diagnosis is made or not long afterwards, suggesting that delays do indeed contribute to poor outcomes. Thomas et al. (2006) state that one of the reasons for poor outcomes in this age group is detection at a later stage, and, according to Albritton and Bleyer (2003: 2589), the time lag between symptom onset and diagnosis for all solid tumours in adolescence (except Hodgkin's disease) increases as age increases.

According to Lewis (2005: 255), there is a widely expressed perception of significant and avoidable delay in the initial diagnosis, but that evidence for this is sparse. Whiteson (2005) also alludes to 'anecdotal' evidence of delays and suggests some of the factors that may contribute to a late diagnosis include: teenagers' reluctance to seek medical advice and their lack of knowledge about symptoms, parents' decreased involvement in their sons' and daughters' health care, lack of experience of cancers in this age group among general practitioners, and the lack of a clear pathway of referral.

Matthew Engel's (2005) account of his 13-year-old son Laurie's diagnosis suggests that there is a deeply embedded cultural resistance to the diagnosis of cancer in young people. Laurie was eventually diagnosed with an admittedly extremely rare soft tissue sarcoma 'rhabdomyosarcoma alveolar'. However, even after his initial surgery for what was assumed to be a rectal abscess, the cancer remained undiagnosed. Engel suggests that misdiagnosis is common, as we can see from the following quote:

> Most children on Ward 15 seemed to have been misdiagnosed. British medical students are told if they see a bird on their lawn, they should presume it's a sparrow, not a lanceolated warbler. Paediatric cancer is rare, and non-specialists don't look for it. ('You know,' one

doctor told me, 'a GP could go through their entire career and never see anything like what Laurie has got.' 'But the surgeon missed it too,' I protested. 'The same' he said.) Several mothers told us they were written off as paranoid, or their children as moaning wimps.

(Engel 2005: 21)

Engel maintains that had Laurie's cancer been picked up sooner or if a sample had been sent for biopsy after his surgery, the disease could have been identified 10 weeks earlier, which might have resulted in his son's survival. Such concerns over diagnosis extend through the whole age range and an example of the upper end of the spectrum is recounted in an article by Jackie Daly, the friend of a young woman called Kelly, who died at 28 from cervical cancer. She had been tested by three different doctors for chlamydia, and despite the fact that all the tests had come back negative, it appears that it was not until months later that the correct diagnosis was made (Daly 2006). It was, as in Matthew Engel's example, apparently a case of assuming the 'bird was a sparrow'. Similarly Peter Cura's cancer of the kidney remained un-diagnosed for well over a year. Although he had sought medical advice at an early stage, his GP had said that at his age (27) it was very unlikely to be cancer. The consultant later told the family that had Peter's kidney been removed 18 months earlier, he would probably have lived (Lacey 2006).

Dr James, the GP at the university health centre where George[1] was a student, referred him early for diagnosis of the osteosarcoma, of which he suspected George's symptoms were indicative. But Dr James pointed out how problematic diagnosis among this age group can be when, for example, an unspecific and potentially lifestyle-related symptom such as 'tiredness' may be all that is presented to the GP. As Dr James said:

> I mustn't be ... critical of colleagues in [asking] ... 'How good is your clinical acumen?' I could easily have been forgiven if I'd sent him [George] away with a non-steroidal anti-inflammatory drug and said, 'Come back in a fortnight if it's not better.' ... he was a guy playing football, no history of trauma, no history of injury or falling, but had got this pain and, and this swelling. Not a very big swelling, just a minimal amount of difference on one side as compared with the other. But it was a difference and it was a bit hot and I was just suspicious ... they are only young and you don't expect them to be developing a cancer, [but] be careful because they do ... And of course you see that [along]side of lots of other people who are tired all the time because they go to bed too late.

The possibility of delayed diagnosis of cancer is not confined to this age group, and in a review of the literature of patients' views of cancer services, Farrell (2006) identifies GP delay in referral as stemming either from a lack of knowledge or the refusal to take the patients' symptoms seriously. Even common cancers such as those of the breast can be misdiagnosed among older women because of, for example, 'unimpressive findings' upon physical examination, negative mammograms, failure to biopsy and delays in referral (Steyskal 1996). However, while delays in diagnosis may take place for a variety of reasons among other older adults, when a teenager or young adult presents symptoms the situation may be compounded by the physician's lack of expectation that a young person will have malignant disease and also the young patient's lack of experience and confidence in pressing for further investigation.

Yet any delay may be aggravated in the first instance by resistance on the part of the young person to seek medical advice. Clearly young adults are not unique in delaying consultation: Smith et al. (2005) show through a meta-ethnographic synthesis that analysed 32 papers on diagnosis, a variety of reasons contribute to presentation delays in the wider population. These include: vague symptoms remaining unrecognized, embarrassment, the fear of being seen as neurotic, fearing the diagnosis of cancer and the gender of the patient – men being less inclined to seek help than women. Farrell (2006) also identifies fear of cancer diagnosis as being a contributory factor in patient delay. Nevertheless, it is likely that not only will these contributory factors be manifested by young people; they will be exacerbated by a lack of awareness of the implications and what Albritton and Bleyer (2003: 2595) refer to as 'inadequate supervision' as parents try to give their son or daughter the 'space' they expect at this age. However proficient a GP becomes in diagnosis, this can only be carried out if symptoms are presented, and it is examples from the fieldwork of patient delays to which we turn first.

In some instances the lack of realization, on the part of the young person, of the potentially serious nature of symptoms may be related to their non-specific nature, but this can be exacerbated by a lack of knowledge about the implications, as indicated by Gemma:

> I had put off going to the GP for months as I thought the swelling in the left side of my neck was due to my wisdom teeth, which had caused me problems for over a year with recurrent flare-ups and infections and was waiting to have them removed. I had been on holiday with my boyfriend for two weeks and the swelling was becoming noticeable on the left side of my neck. I was only worried at the time about being unwell on holiday. I returned to work after my holiday and had thought about going to the dentist to get another check-up and most likely another round of antibiotics. I didn't find the time and had what I considered more important things to do and I am not one for taking time off work for any illness. My teeth were in no pain and so I left it.
>
> (Gemma)

Despite the fact that Gemma was a trained nurse (working on an orthopaedic ward), she rationalized the symptoms as trivial and was concerned primarily about her holiday with her boyfriend and other activities that demanded her attention.

In addition to a tendency to dismiss worrying symptoms in the belief that they can be explained by minor medical conditions, there are also cases in which symptoms may even be viewed with pleasure, for example, weight loss. Weight consciousness and a desire to be thin may be found particularly among young women. Brannen et al. (1994) document that 46 per cent of young women have tried to lose weight within the previous year, and in Devika's account we can see that her weight loss was welcome and the symptoms were thought trivial by the GP:

> At first, we [my family] didn't even know I had cancer, I was just thin, which I liked, a bit pale and sick quite a bit of the time. When I went to the doctors they just said it was an infection – nothing to worry about. So we just ignored it and I got on with my normal life, which, without me knowing, was soon coming to an end.
>
> (Devika)

Philip had experienced rectal bleeding for a considerable time before family and friends, in whom he eventually confided, insisted that he seek a medical opinion. He described his reluctance to seek medical advice as follows:

> For just over a year I'd been passing blood through my back passage and never thought anything of it, I thought, oh, it'll pass, kind of thing, at one point it started getting a bit worse and I spoke to my mother and she said, 'Get to the doctor's.' I left it for a bit longer ... Then I spoke to the receptionist at work and she said the same, she said, 'You'd better go.' She forced me to go to a doctor's from work. Anyhow I went and he examined me and it all went from there really. About two weeks after I'd been to the doctor's, I was told it was cancer ... I felt fine, I didn't feel ill or anything ... They reckon I'd had it about four years or something like that.
>
> (Philip)

Here the diagnosis followed quickly after the initial consultation, which had been delayed by Philip's reluctance to acknowledge that the symptoms might be serious. The reluctance to admit to such symptoms and to seek medical help is not confined to young adults (Farrell 2006), yet to ignore the problem for more than a year might be considered an unusually lengthy period. This may have been because Philip 'felt fine', indeed, as a trainee Outward Bound instructor he would have been 'fit' if not healthy, and at some level probably did not believe that he could have a cancer so rare among this age group.

Later in this chapter we shall see the account of Mark's diagnosis with testicular cancer, yet here it is worth noting here that it was only because of Mark's own diagnosis that an acquaintance of his sought medical advice when he too manifested symptoms. As Mark said:

> There's a lad down the road ... and he's had testicular cancer. He said he would never, ever have gone to the doctor's as fast as he did [it was] because of knowing somebody who was that young having something like that.
>
> (Mark)

Yet Mark acknowledges his own ignorance before his diagnosis despite the fact that his father had the same disease diagnosed when he had been 40:

> I feel that nobody talked to me [about cancer] ... I thought you had to be 40 to get cancer ... I thought you had to be a lot older. When they told me testicular cancer was most common between 13 and 25 [I was really surprised] nobody had ever mentioned that.
>
> (Mark)

Some of the cancers were diagnosed almost by accident; it was only chance that led Adrian, an apprentice of 18, to seek medical treatment for an injury as he had been unaware of any worrying symptoms:

> It was lucky that I actually come across it, because I was at work and I had an accident ... I cut my testicle sac, and I went to the accident and emergency and they said, 'We'll stitch you up and then we'll send you for a scan.' And that's when they picked it up, so they said if I hadn't had the accident, I wouldn't have found out about it.
>
> (Adrian)

Emma's diagnosis was made after a routine consultation for what had been assumed to be a cyst. The diagnosis did not follow swiftly causing an initial delay, but the majority of the delay in her treatment stemmed from her reluctance to accept the fact she had cancer:

> I missed appointments ... because I didn't think it was going to be anything bad. They told me it wasn't. I thought I was just going back for a check-up after my operation. They'd already told me ... I said, 'Am I going to have cancer?' because some more people in my family have got cancer as well. And she said, 'No, definitely not.' And I did

... [but] I couldn't believe it ... they told me the beginning of the year but, no, I couldn't believe it. I wanted to not have any treatment. I wanted to delay it for ages so I'd have my hair for longer ... nobody told me what it was going to do to me. They just told me I had cancer, they didn't tell me the side effects or anything.

(Emma)

Emma continued by saying that she still found it almost impossible to believe that she had cancer but had eventually agreed to treatment. While in these accounts it appears to have been the young people who did not recognize the symptoms, who delayed seeking medical advice or who could not accept the diagnosis, the majority of delays were related to GPs' lack of recognition of the potentially serious nature of the symptoms. Some of the young men in the study had been keen athletes before their illnesses and were used to having sports injuries, and this contributed to misdiagnoses in the early stages. At the age of 16 and still at school, Luke's osteosarcoma was initially thought to have been a sports injury:

I did quite a lot of football, like on Sunday leagues and stuff like that and I just thought it was a natural injury due to football. I had the problem round about Christmas time and I had it for about four months or so. And I kept going back to the doctor's but they just kept giving me pills like co-codamol and stuff, but it didn't really work. That's when I went to hospital and they found out I had the cancer.

(Luke)

Luke's aunt was visiting at the time of the interview and contributed the following observations:

Because Gill [Luke's mum] is a nurse, she had him there [at the GPs] ... but she couldn't get them to send Luke for an X-ray or a scan or to do any blood tests or anything ... They just continually put it down to a sports injury even though it was evident that the medication wasn't working ... and also his loss of weight and his not eating and pain ... She [his mother] knew there was something [wrong] earlier on but couldn't get anybody to take any notice. I think that was from her point of view, certainly ... the worst time ... Once it was recognized, when somebody says 'Do this, that and the other', it lessens the burden in a way, psychologically because you feel that somebody else is on your side whereas when nobody will take any notice you're just battling on your own.

(Luke's aunt)

Aidan, close in age to Luke, also had osteosarcoma that was similarly mis-diagnosed. He had been a keen sports player, and as his mother observed, she felt that this could have contributed to the delay in the recognition of both his cancer and that of others in the age group:

> I think that's why diagnosis is often delayed in young teenagers. Because doctors don't look for cancer . . . which is fair enough. So in their career they might only ever see two cases, if that. I think the diagnosis is a bit of a problem really. We did have to battle with doctors backwards and forwards. And it's only really because a friend of ours is a consultant that we were suddenly shifted forward and got the MRI scan and everything quite fast.
>
> (Aidan's mother)

Yet another osteosarcoma was misdiagnosed as a sports injury when Hoody, an athlete hoping to be included in the 2012 Olympics, manifested knee problems:

> Well, I went for months and months thinking it was an injury which I started off noticing as a pain when I was hit in the back of the leg with a football. And quite a hard knock, had a bit of a lump that day and, you know, noticed knee pains for a time after that . . . it got a bit worse, then one of my friends who I was doing a course with had a knee problem and he said, 'Why don't you go and see the doctor?' I left it a few weeks and then I went and he diagnosed it as bursitis which is a knee injury. And then I was referred for physio where they did a lot of short wave therapy . . . for a few weeks . . . it all fitted the diagnosis you know . . . I saw two GPs who didn't see anything and two physios as well. My mum was asking for X-rays at the physio's for ages but, you know, they just were saying, 'Oh, it's this knee injury.' I mean, the physios didn't check it out or anything. But apparently physios can't order X-rays but that would have shown the cancer, but they didn't do that. I mean, that just delays it even more, allowed it to spread to my lungs and cause even more problems. I just think that an X-ray or something like is fairly simple . . . apparently you can ask for your own X-rays which I wish we'd done in the end . . . it was really convincing what they were saying but, you know, I didn't understand why I was in so much pain. But they just kept going with the same treatment. And I didn't feel any different. And they said, 'Oh, no, it's helping, it's nothing.' But short wave would have just made the tumour grow even more because it's influencing the cells to grow. So they eventually said it might be cartilage problem. And they nearly gave me a cortisone injection into it, but I was too young,

> luckily. I mean, if I was old enough they would have given me that
> and that would have caused many problems, so many problems.
>
> (Hoody)

Again we see a mother wanting further investigation but being placated with
reassurances. After consulting two GPs and having had treatment from two
physiotherapists, Hoody had treated his knee himself with ice packs and the
swelling had subsided sufficiently for him to be able to travel to a diving
course in the Philippines. However, while he was there, his condition worsened. The doctor attending him did not divulge his concerns to Hoody, but
in a telephone call to his parents, who were in the UK, the doctor revealed his
suspicion that osteosarcoma was the cause of Hoody's pain.

Ross's osteosarcoma first manifested as a lump on the back of his hand.
He sought medical advice at an early stage but the chance of it being a malignancy was thought so remote that the eventual diagnosis was not made for
five months:

> A lump appeared on the back of my left hand on the third meta-
> carpal. And I didn't really know why it had appeared. Anyway a few
> weeks had passed, and and it hadn't gone down which I had ex-
> pected it would have done. So I went to the hospital to have it looked
> at, and they X-rayed it. And initially they thought it was a break in
> the bone that had healed and sort of kept growing, or it [might have
> been] an infection of the bone ... after I ... had a couple of X-rays,
> they said, 'Come back in a month's time and we'll X-ray you again
> and see if there's any change.' And he said then that there is a pos-
> sibility it could be cancer but we really don't think it will be. They
> said, you know it's virtually no chance it will be. So they weren't too
> concerned.
>
> (Ross)

Ross attributed the lack of concern to his age and said that because he was
only 22, the doctors assumed the lump was not likely to be malignant.
However, by the time it had been diagnosed, there had been a spread to Ross's
lungs.

Lucy, still at school, was interviewed in the ward with her mother at her
bedside. They spoke of the early stages of the illness when her mother, although not medically qualified, believed that Lucy's heartbeat sounded different from usual and as a consequence took her to the doctor. She said the
following about her attempt to persuade medical professionals that she wasn't
simply being over-anxious:

I felt like a paranoid mother, but, you know how sometimes you sort of cuddle up on the bed? I'd say things, 'Your heart's beating', she'd say, 'That's good.' And it normally has a very hollow drum-like sound, but it sounded more muffled ... it was obviously because I could hear it through the tumour [that] was developing and it was affecting the sound ... There's a neighbour who's a nurse and I said, 'Is it something to be worried about?' [she said] probably not but it was half-term the following week ... and she said, just take her in and ask the doctor to have a listen. And she [the doctor] said a flow murmur is quite common in young girls because the blood could be going round at quite a rate.

(Lucy's mother)

Lucy's mother said that she had spoken to other mothers on the ward who had experienced similar difficulties with their concerns not being taken seriously by their doctors. Lucy said the following about her diagnosis:

It started off with back pain. I thought it was just because I fell over, and then it just seemed to get worse and worse. And when I went to the doctor she said that it was just muscle pain. And my mum had noticed that my heart beat didn't sound normal. So she asked her to look at that, and they said it was a flow murmur ... And then I went back a week later about the back pain again. They said it was still just muscle pain and still having flow murmurs. And then a couple of weeks later I went back to the doctor's again but this time because it was a cough ... and it was every time that I lay down ... so the doctor thought it might have been a chest infection. So he rang up [the hospital] and wrote a note to A&E saying that he thought it was a chest infection.

(Lucy)

The severe stomach pains that were symptomatic of Charlotte's liver cancer were originally thought by her and her family to be related to her periods. As her grandmother, present at the interview, said, they all thought she was being 'a bit melodramatic'. However, when the pains became worse and medical opinion was sought, the cancer was misdiagnosed first as an abscess, then as gallstones. After four months Charlotte was transferred to a specialist unit where cancer was diagnosed. Neither Charlotte nor her grandmother were sure if her age had contributed to the amount of time the correct diagnosis took, but it was clear that cancer had been far from their minds as a possibility.

James began to have headaches and blurred vision, accompanied by extreme tiredness. He eventually presented these symptoms to his GP who diagnosed blocked sinuses. When his prescribed medication failed to take effect, he went back to the surgery where he saw a different doctor who asked him to read the wall chart which he 'could not even see', he was then sent to the eye clinic at the local hospital – a cancer diagnosis still far from everyone's minds:

> The doctor did some tests but did not know what was wrong ... a couple of days later I saw an eye consultant and he noticed I had pools of fluid behind my eyes. The doctors wondered if there might be a serious situation and decided that I should have a CT scan ... [and] blood tests.
>
> (James)

The results of James' tests revealed that he had ALL (acute lymphoblastic leukaemia) but, like Emma, he refused to believe it and when the doctor attempted to tell him more about his condition he said, 'I was too distraught to take it in.'

It is unclear whether any of the delays in diagnosis affected the outcomes for the young people discussed thus far. However, one of the participants, Michelle, interviewed with her mother, suggested that the GP's early reluctance to acknowledge that she might have a potentially serious condition had resulted in her eventually being diagnosed with an adrenal tumour at a late stage. Michelle begins her account by recalling the early manifestations of her illness at the age of 18:

> Well, I had high blood pressure ... when I was about 18. They diagnosed me with high blood pressure ... at the time before I started putting the weight on. Then whilst I was going to the gym I was putting weight on instead of losing it ... but then I just thought, well, maybe your muscle is building up underneath your fat or something like that.
>
> (Michelle)

Having been put on medication for high blood pressure that she was told she would need to take for the rest of her life, Michelle determined to get herself fit by exercising in the gym, though she could not understand why she was still putting on weight. She rationalized the weight gain and though no explanation for her high blood pressure had been offered, she assumed that she was being well cared for by her GP. Michelle then embarked upon a degree at her local university but endured ill health throughout her course. However, on the assumption that her health would improve if she kept herself fit, she kept exercising and using the gym. Her health continued to present many problems that she attributed to stress, particularly as her health worsened during her final degree exams. When Michelle eventually had hospital treatment, it appears that the doctors found it hard to believe that no tests had been carried out to determine the cause of her high blood pressure. Michelle's mother, present at the interview, contributed the following comment on the delayed diagnosis:

> All the things that Michelle had, like, she put on weight and they call it moon face, and she sort of ballooned out with her face and lost all her neck and that is all the symptoms of it. But because you don't understand these things you think it's just, you know . . . if I think, I can still get really angry that they didn't take the high blood pressure at 18 any further than they did, because there's not many young people that get [it] you know, she came home and she just said the doctor says I've got to take tablets for the rest of my life for high blood pressure.
>
> (Michelle's mother)

The prognosis for Michelle was unclear, but both she and her mother were of the opinion that had she been diagnosed with the adrenal tumour three years earlier, she would have stood a better chance of recovery. Doctors might not be 'looking for cancer' in a young adult, but in Michelle's case an unusual symptom had been diagnosed. High blood pressure is not common in this age group, yet this was treated symptomatically rather than its underlying cause being investigated as sinister.

At the older end of the age range, Kelly at 26 also experienced a delay in her diagnosis. In her case, the situation was complicated by a combination of her unspecific symptoms and the fact that she had recently given birth. The lengthy quote that follows indicates the delays and her frustration:

> I had quite a difficult birth and then after it suffered post-traumatic stress syndrome, so I had to be put on medication for that. And then I felt these lumps in my neck . . . and I've always thought if you ever have any lumps on your neck, always get them checked out. So I went to the doctor's and he had a feel . . . and he said it could have been a number of things. I think one of his diagnoses was it could be flu . . . but I think I would have known if I had flu, wouldn't I? Anyway they sent me for some blood [tests] and they said, 'Come back in a month, blah, blah . . .' So that's what I did. But I started to get more [tired] and I mean I was working at the time as well and I had the little one. And I did start to feel more tired but I just put it down to having a child, you know, running round after them. Anyway I kept going back for blood tests, you know back and forth for blood tests for five months. And eventually I went to see him and

he says, 'Right, your blood tests have come back', and there was something not right in my blood. And he said, 'How do you feel?' He says, 'Do you feel unwell?' And I says, 'Yes', I mean, I kept going but I felt as if I stopped and really thought about it, I could have been really ill, do you know what I mean? So he says, 'Right, well, we'll refer you to the ear, nose and throat specialist.' So I went up there and he shoved in one of them endoscopy things ... it was horrific, horrible ... oh, it was nasty. And he said he couldn't find anything, so he asked for a biopsy. So that was the next week actually. I was quite surprised. He says, 'I'm going to book you in next week.' ... So I went down there and had a lump taken out, awake. Cutting through gristle, it was horrible, you know I could hear it all and, oh, nasty. And then it was really quick, because it had taken so long and then everything happened so quick ... I had an appointment to go and see him again in a fortnight. So that was it really ... I personally feel initially I was fobbed off a lot by the doctor ... don't get me wrong, I do like my doctor but I did feel as though he'd messed about a bit ... I mean, we eventually got there but I think he could have maybe taken it a bit more seriously. But there again it is a busy surgery, they have that many patients ... I think he basically thought it might just go away, you know. Because he said, 'Oh, it could be viral you know', or like I say, I could have had flu and, he was just giving me all these excuses ... but for some reason I just knew there was something there. I mean, I didn't think it was cancer, but I knew there was something not right. But I felt he did fob me off a lot and I was getting quite frustrated towards the end ... I was quite tempted to get a second opinion before he referred me.

(Kelly)

Several issues are raised by Kelly's account. First, at the slightly older age of 26 she was aware that a lump in the neck should be taken seriously and presented quickly, but while concerned that she had something more serious than flu, she still did not expect it to be cancer. Clearly the doctor did not expect a cancer diagnosis either, and perhaps too easily attributed her symptoms to postnatal tiredness or depression perhaps because Kelly had experienced post-traumatic stress after the birth. Nevertheless, despite Kelly's concerns, she was still apparently unable to progress the situation for five months, but it is interesting that Kelly makes excuses for the delays by referring to the busy nature of the practice and the amount of pressure the doctor was under.

In contrast to the delays discussed thus far, there were also examples of early recognition by the GP. Craig, who presented a testicular lump to his GP, was referred for specialist investigation immediately; Marc too was treated early for his testicular cancer. In these cases the illness, testicular cancer, may be both more easily identifiable symptomatically and more readily associated with the age group and as a result more likely to be picked up. Indeed, in Craig's case, his doctor told him that it was 'pretty common in my age group'. However, in Mark's case he believed his testicular cancer had been diagnosed early because his father too had been diagnosed with the illness. While this had resulted in his own enhanced awareness, as we saw earlier in this chapter, Mark had still regarded the cancer as one of older age. However, he said he felt the speed with which he saw the specialist reflected his GP's increased concern over the family link:

> The doctor seemed pretty relaxed about it, said it could have been a cyst, it could have been numerous things … but [he] never, ever mentioned the cancer word … I went to see a specialist about seven or eight days later. [I] got through rather quickly but I don't think it [usually] happens just like that.
>
> (Mark)

While there was no delay in Thomas's diagnosis of osteosarcoma, this was not because the symptoms were recognized by his GP, who had thought the osteosarcoma was a benign cyst. Nevertheless, it was investigated at a relatively early stage because his mother took him directly to A&E:

> I was struggling to walk … I was just limping and I was walking home with my friends at night and I couldn't really keep up with them, I had to keep asking them to wait for me and eventually it got too much to walk on, so my Mum took me to the GP, first of all, and he had a look at it and he thought it was what's called a Baker's cyst underneath my knee that had burst so I left it for a while but I still couldn't walk on it so my Mum took me into the [hospital] and they thought it was the same thing but they did an X-ray … and they saw like a black mark on the X-ray where my knee was, so they kept me in overnight, did a few scans and everything and that's when they started to find out about what it could be so that was a bit shocking really … [The GP] was really surprised afterwards … He never thought [it was] that, I mean, you don't think of that though, do you? I mean, pain in the knee it could be anything, a muscle cramp or anything, you don't suddenly think it's cancer.
>
> (Thomas)

A similarly swift diagnosis was made of Ricky's leukaemia, but as Sue, Lead Macmillan Clinical Nurse Specialist for teenagers and young adults points out:

> Leukaemias and lymphomas are the ones diagnosed the fastest as they are very sick, very quickly and will have the outward appearances of being ill, i.e. lumps, bruises, feeling very tired and looking pale. They are also diagnosed with a blood test – which is very simple, cheap and easy.
>
> (Sue)

Toni, a young woman with ambitions to be a nurse, was diagnosed quickly with Hodgkin's disease. Her symptoms were taken seriously from the outset perhaps because this is a condition associated with the age group:

> I had a lump on my neck and I'd had it before, but it'd just gone down after a couple of days and [then] it just didn't go down. So I went to a doctor and it was all very rushed, he was fascinated. He was looking at it and measuring and ... and prodding and then the next day he referred me to ear, nose and throat people and they did all the checks and that.
>
> (Toni)

Despite Hodgkin's disease being comparatively common in the age group, its relative frequency does not mean that young people will associate a lump in the neck with anything serious or life-threatening. Indeed, they may not even know what 'Hodgkin's disease' is when it is diagnosed as shown in Steven's account:

> This lump came in my neck, I went and had it removed ... you presume it's going to be something and nothing ... mum said, 'Do you want me to come down to hospital?' I said, 'Oh, no, no, it's all right, no panic, no, I'll give you a ring later on.' So fair enough, [I] went down, [I] can't remember the name of the doctor who was my surgeon, but anyway a nice bloke. Sat me down and said to me 'You've got Hodgkin's disease.' Now to me you might as well have just talked in Swahili, I hadn't got a clue what he meant. I thought, 'Oh, all right, yes, big deal, give me a course of antibiotics, I'll see you in a week.' And it was odd really because he wouldn't tell me it was cancer ... I had to start pushing a little bit for that ... the treatment, he said was ... chemotherapy ... and I'd heard of that, I knew sort of what that was. And that's when it sort of hit home a little bit.
>
> (Steven)

This extract raises a number of issues, at 18, Steven – a heavy goods mechanic – would be unlikely to wish for or to expect his mother to accompany him to a hospital appointment even though she had offered to go with him. Her offer is unsurprising as previous research among the parents of young adults with cancer shows that mothers in particular find it hard to relinquish responsibility and involvement in their young adult sons' and daughters' health – Steven's rejection of the offer is equally unsurprising (Grinyer 2002a). Despite his understandable wish to be independent, when given the diagnosis, Steven seemingly had little understanding of the implications. As he said, the diagnosis might as well have been in Swahili. Here we see the 'in between' stage of life resulting in being old enough to attend such appointments alone, without necessarily having the knowledge to interpret the encounter. Despite Steven's mother not being at the consultation, she was the first person he contacted and she went straight to the hospital:

> My head just went then and I couldn't really think anything ... Like head went, legs didn't work, just complete shock ... I don't know whether it's normal or not ... So I rang my mother at work, she only worked round the corner, so she came round. She spoke to a nurse for a short period and then spoke to the doctor, and then came in to see me ... They got upset, my mum more than my dad ... my mum was always there and she'd go to any hospital appointment I had or read up and tell me about, tell me about stuff because she's a nurse ... which in some ways helped.
>
> (Steven)

It might be thought surprising, as Steven's mother was a nurse, that she had not been at the consultation from the outset – she might even have feared that the lump in his neck signified a serious condition. However, when we consider Steven's age, we can see that his preference to be on his own was predictable for a young man of this age, but it is interesting to note that subsequently it seems to have been his mother who acted as the interface between Steven and the medical staff in terms of reading up about the illness and passing the information on to him, thus he was relinquishing some of his early bid for independence.

The early diagnosis of cancers may relate to them having been previously seen by practitioners in the primary care setting. This may be more likely at a university medical practice where, once a cancer has been diagnosed in this age group, it becomes more likely that subsequent cases will be recognized as potentially serious and followed up with more urgency. In a discussion with George's mother, Helen, she said the following about George's diagnosis with osteosarcoma while he was a student away from home in his first year at university:

> George's diagnosis was handled very well by the university practice that had had previous experience of an osteosarcoma. He had a sore

knee in March which was initially assumed by the doctor to be a sports injury. But when his symptoms did not improve he went back for a second appointment in May and at this consultation his condition was immediately recognized as serious. He went straight from the clinic to the hospital for an X-ray and even before George was told the diagnosis, the GP had booked a bed in a specialist bone cancer unit.

(Helen)

After his second consultation with the university GP, George was diagnosed within 24 hours. The only way in which Helen felt the process might have been expedited was if rather than George having to take the initiative to make a second appointment – which he did primarily because his knee problem prevented him from playing football – a second appointment a month later could have been made automatically. This could have been cancelled if George had recovered, but would have removed the onus from him having to seek further advice.

Discussion

We began this chapter with reference to Lewis (2005) and Whiteson (2005) who both refer to a lack of evidence to support their strong suspicions that late diagnosis and delays are a particular problem in young adult cancers. Yet it seems from the evidence presented here that there are indeed certain age-specific barriers that make the early presentation and diagnosis of symptoms less likely and are closely related to Whiteson's list of contributory factors. Such delays can contribute to poor outcomes and this is indeed a serious issue.

Young adulthood is a life stage that brings with it a separation from dependency on parents in many ways. This includes an understandable tendency to be private over health-related issues. This may be the case particularly if symptoms relate to parts of the body about which young people feel uncomfortable discussing with a parent, for example, testicular or breast lumps or gynaecological symptoms. While breast cancer may be rare in this age group, the link between sexually transmitted infections and carcinoma of the cervix and uterus makes these cancers relatively frequent (Birch et al. 2003). And according to Selby et al. (2005), the incidence of testicular cancer is increasing.

Additionally, the young person may not have the knowledge to recognize early symptoms as being potentially serious or life-threatening and as a result will delay seeking advice; this can be exacerbated by the fact that they do not wish their plans to be disrupted. We can see in Gemma's case that she did not take her symptoms seriously, nor was she willing to allow them to disrupt her plans to go on holiday or get on with building her career. Clearly it is not only young adults who delay seeking advice (Smith et al. 2005) – to make such an assumption would be to idealize the health-related behaviour of older adults while pathologizing that of the younger adults. However, in older adults, the delay may result from a fear of cancer, while among the younger age group the possibility of cancer is less likely to be recognized – indeed, we have seen examples of the disbelief that can result from the diagnosis.

So even when advice has been sought, the diagnosis may be rejected as in Emma's example or the implications may not be clear. Given the likelihood of a parent not being present at an initial consultation, this can result in a situation where, as in Steven's case, he had no clear understanding of the meaning of the diagnosis. In general, being accompanied by a supporter can be helpful to any consultation where a diagnosis of serious illness may be made, and such support may be more likely with either much younger or much older patients who take a parent, partner or friend with them.

However, the majority of the delays were caused not by a lack of willingness to seek medical advice, but by reassurance from a professional – too readily accepted – that the symptoms were not serious. It seems that Engel's (2005) observation that the medical assumption of the 'bird being a sparrow rather than a lanceolated warbler' has been borne out in many of the accounts presented above. Many GPs will not have seen a case in their surgery, so when vague or imprecise symptoms are presented that can be interpreted as muscle strain, a sports injury or simply tiredness due to too many late nights and partying, this seems a much more likely diagnosis. Indeed, it is a much more likely diagnosis in the majority of cases and as a result it may even seem alarmist for a GP presented with such symptoms to assume a more serious cause and worry the young person unduly by ordering what may turn out to be unnecessary, distressing and expensive tests.

If cancer in teenagers and young adults is increasing (Birch 2005; Selby et al. 2005; Thomas et al. 2006), it is important to raise awareness among all those concerned in diagnosis and treatment. Education programmes on the issue for young people coupled with primary care practitioners having an enhanced awareness, that, though still relatively rare, there are more cancers in the ages 15–24 than in children 0–15 (Albritton and Bleyer 2003; Birch et al. 2003; Whiteson 2005) may combine to lead to earlier diagnoses. However, one of the challenges of achieving increased awareness is a need to balance this against causing alarm and subjecting young people to a battery of unnecessary tests for non-serious illness. There are likely to be occasions when errors are made on both sides, but the application of the precautionary principle can be justified in such a potentially high risk scenario when failure to diagnose early enough can result in death. Health services at schools, universities, colleges and other establishments where there is a high concentration of young people may benefit from clear guidelines relating in particular to those cancers, such as osteosarcoma, found in the age group that may be hard to distinguish from routine conditions such as sporting injuries. A parallel raising of awareness among the young people may also be effective in encouraging them to seek medical advice at an earlier stage.

At a time when guidelines (NICE 2005a) for services for teenagers and young adults with cancer are the focus of policy-making, these are issues that need to be recognized and embedded into any planning for future provision if teenagers and young adults with cancer are to stand the best chance of survival. Further implications for policy and practice are discussed in greater detail in Chapter 8.

Key points

Delays in diagnosis occur because of:

- primary care practitioners not looking for cancer in this age group;

- symptoms being vague and ambiguous;

- statistical likelihood of malignancy;

- young adults' lack of awareness;

- young adults' lack of motivation/willingness to seek medical advice;

- young adults' reluctance to accept a cancer diagnosis;

- parents relinquishing responsibility for their son or daughter's health.

More rapid diagnosis is made when:

- more common cancers are presented;

- young adult is informed and aware;

- physician has dealt with similar cases;

- symptoms are presented to a hospital A&E department.

Note

1   Please see the Foreword for details of George and the role he and his parents played in the instigation of this research.

3 Settings of care

Fundamental to the NICE Guidance (2005a) on cancer services for adolescents and young adults is an acknowledgment that an appropriate setting of care is important and that a staff trained in the needs of the age group is of central importance to such provision. This document, at least in part, stems from increasing debate over who should care for teenagers and young adults with cancer.

The hazards of inappropriate care and the dangers of falling between paediatric and adult services are addressed by Albritton and Bleyer (2003) who quote from Leonard et al.'s UK study:

> Adult oncologists may be 'untutored in arranging ancillary medical, psychological and educational supports that are so important to people who are facing dangerous diseases and taxing treatments at a vulnerable time in their lives' and 'unpracticed in managing rare sarcomas,' whereas paediatric oncologists may 'have little to no experience in epithelial tumours or some of the other tumours common in late adolescence'.
>
> (Albritton and Bleyer 2003: 2590)

According to Whiteson (2005: 3), 'cancer services are delivered by an out-of-date infrastructure that, by and large, fails teenagers and young adults'. Whiteson also claims that adult and paediatric services do not cooperate well and have different protocols for the same diseases. This raises the question of 'Who should care for young people with cancer?' The problem is addressed through contributions from a range of professionals including: a paediatric oncologist, an adult oncologist, an adolescent unit nurse, a paediatric nurse, an adult nurse and a social worker (Arbuckle et al. 2005). These authors come to the conclusion that 'Shared disease expertise and increasing knowledge of the psychosocial needs of young people, delivered within an age-appropriate environment, is likely to produce the best outcomes for young people' (2005: 239). Yet despite such opinion and the NICE Guidance (2005a), the nature and location of the optimum care setting have continued to generate controversy. As Arbuckle et al. say, there has been much discussion between paediatric and adult oncologists about who is best qualified to care for the age group and Lewis (2005) and Morgan and Hubber (2004), themselves professionals working within specialist Teenage Cancer Trust (TCT) wards, all report evidence of some resistance to age-specific units.

There is an argument that disease-specific centres may offer the best setting of care. However, Arbuckle et al. (2005: 235) maintain that while care in a non-age-specific environment *may* be delivered by staff who enjoy looking after adolescents, it may equally be given by those who fear contact with the age group because they feel intimidated, inadequate or are simply indifferent. These authors also suggest that adolescents may be regarded by staff as no different than adults, but the founding principle of this volume – and also of the NICE Guidance (2005a) is that young adults are a distinct group with specific needs, and this is the basis of the philosophy of the TCT wards situated at a limited number of hospitals in the UK (in 2006, 7 had been established, 10 were in development and 15 were in discussion: Source: TCT website 2006b).

Nevertheless, as we saw in Chapter 1, defining the needs of an age group around which it is difficult to draw boundaries and which encompasses a range of life experiences is difficult. Thus, in order to ensure that age-specific care is experienced as appropriate across the spectrum in ways that complement and support medical treatment, it is essential to understand from the young people's perspective how services are perceived, which aspects of a variety of care settings are found to be supportive and appropriate and, conversely, what is experienced as unacceptable; otherwise there can be no understanding of what an 'appropriate' setting means in practice. Indeed, it may be that no single definition of 'appropriate care' can capture all the needs of a disparate group of young people.

The participants in this study had been treated in a variety of different care environments, thus we are able to take a range of experience into account. To some extent the care setting appeared to be related to where the young people lived at the time of diagnosis and their consequent geographical proximity to a specialist adolescent cancer facility, of which there are a limited number. Some participants had been treated in several hospitals with differing facilities and so were able to offer some comparisons between the specialist and non-specialist environments.

The care settings experienced included: children's wards, general wards and cancer wards largely occupied by the elderly, through to the specialist facilities offered by Teenage Cancer Trust wards and other cancer treatment centres with young people's units. In some cases the hospital was near home, friends and family, in others it was located some distance away in a specialist centre. All these factors are addressed through an analysis of the interview material in terms of the impact place of care had upon the young adults' experiences.

The non-specialist care setting

The following accounts make it clear that the setting in which treatment takes place has a profound effect on young adults and teenagers. We begin with Michelle, a young woman of 21 who had been treated in a number of different wards and hospitals, none of which specialized in teenage and adolescent care and in which she had both positive and negative experiences. Michelle had at first been placed on an assessment ward in a non-specialist centre:

> I had one night in there ... [I] couldn't get to sleep in there because there was a woman screaming and shouting, I got no sleep at all. I wanted my mum to stay with me; I would not let her leave because I was so scared. So I made her sleep in a chair next to me.
>
> (Michelle)

Clearly Michelle found this environment frightening and the fact that she wanted her mother to stay by her bedside reminds us that even at 21, after graduating from university and having attained some independence, the combination of the illness and the strangeness of the care setting had the effect of Michelle needing her mother's presence just as a much younger child might. Yet we should not be surprised at this as Woodgate's (2006: 127) study shows, 'adolescents especially felt protected when their family members were there to watch over them' in hospital.

Mark had been treated on a general men's ward; like Michelle, he was 21 but was married. He too needed support – in his case that of his wife and he had been very anxious that he should be able to secure a private room:

> I was very nervous I didn't want my wife to leave me. On the letter that came it said I could pay for my own private room. And I rang up and I couldn't get through, and my wife and my mother-in-law said to me, you might be better with people round you rather than sat in a room being miserable. So I decided just to go to the hospital and see what happened. And as it happened fortunately they had a room spare ... [but] I didn't want to stop, I wanted to be home, I would have come home the same day if I could have done, but they persuaded me to stop.
>
> (Mark)

For Mark, the issue of age-appropriate care was not significant as his primary concern was to have a private room; not only did he not want to be treated alongside other young adults, he did not want to be in any type of ward. This he attributed to the nature of his cancer:

> I didn't really want to inter-mingle with anybody apart from my family. A single room for me was an absolute blessing because it was my testes. If it had been a lump in my arm, or in my chest or a lump on my foot, yes, of course, I'd love to be with other people to talk to my own age, but because it was something personal I went through a small period of 'was I a man?' Having the testicle removed ... that really upset me ... it was scary.
>
> (Mark)

It seems that Mark would have valued the support of other young people had his cancer been of any other type, yet given that testicular cancer is one of the more common in young adult men, had he been in a specialist environment, he could have received beneficial peer support, and the knowledge that other young men were facing the same fears might have been of reassurance to him during that period when he questioned his masculinity.

Mark felt that the general ward had been the right place for him largely because of the privacy he was given, but a very different experience is re-counted by Michelle. After her distressing night on the assessment ward, she was moved to the general ward of a different hospital, and, like Mark, given her own room. However, her experience there was distressing:

> The fire alarm went off one night. And you're in your own room and I couldn't walk at this stage, it was just after my operation. And I didn't have a clue what was happening, and I thought, well, I don't want to ring my buzzer because I bet everybody's ringing the buzzer and there's only three nurses on through the night, and so they'll be running round telling everybody what's happening, not to panic and stuff. And then nobody came to me for absolutely ages. And so I didn't know what to do, I didn't know whether to panic or what.
>
> (Michelle)

Here, Michelle was in a single room, usually something sought after as in Mark's case. However, on this ward her mother was not present and the fear she felt is clear. As both Michelle's negative experiences took place on wards not specializing in the care of young adults, it might be tempting to attribute her distress solely to this factor. However, of her stay in yet another general ward, Michelle said the following:

> There were a couple of younger people in but I was always the youngest on there ... It was just old ladies ... White curly hair, that's

all you could see ... I mean, some of them were alright but, I mean, most of the time ... they were senile who I was stuck next to. They didn't know what they were talking about, they didn't speak to you. Some of them ... were OK. It's entertaining as well watching them all day do what they do ... I really enjoyed being on the ward ... that's just the normal ward in hospital, but I think that's mainly because I got on really well with all the nurses ... So I liked it on there ... it might just have been because of the nurses, I don't know.

(Michelle)

In contrast to her traumatic night on the assessment ward, and her scare in the side room, Michelle had been quite happy on the general ward largely as a result of her good relationship with the nursing staff. The terms 'enjoy' and 'like' are used in relationship to her stay in hospital, thus suggesting that whatever the setting of care, staff can change the quality of the experience if they relate to the younger patient in an age-appropriate manner. The side room on the cancer unit where Michelle was treated later also offered her the chance to get to know another patient; even though she was a lot older, Michelle appears to have struck up a good relationship with her:

Then I was on the [cancer] unit, when I was on one of the side rooms, it was a room where you could share, just two people in a room ... I was with this lady before they moved me to a room on my own, for about two or three days ... she couldn't believe how positive I was. She thought I was amazing. She was always chatting away to me, she was really nice. So, I mean, you meet, you meet all these people and there's some of them are like really nice, you know, it'd be nice to keep in touch with them.

(Michelle)

So in Michelle's case, we see that of the different non-specialist settings, two were experienced as acceptable and positive. However, other examples show how this age group are on the cusp of services that may be experienced as inappropriate. Craig said that he was treated alongside 'old blokes who slept the majority of the time' but like Michelle, he said that 'the nurses were nice' and that this had made a difference to him. However, Steven's experience of being treated with older people and the alternative prospect of a children's ward suggests a contrasting attitude and quality of experience:

Bit awkward at times 'cause, like, what do you talk about? You know, it's like, 'Well, I went, I went into town on Friday, what did you do'? 'Oh, well, I sat in front of the telly and did me knitting.' I don't have trouble really talking to people ... but when you're in there for hours on end, it's like, well, now what do I talk about? You know people in their sixties and seventies aren't really that interested in fast cars and what I do for a living . . . they've done their living, they've retired and they're pottering around in the garden. But to me it'd be nice to go somewhere where you can talk, you get to talk to nurses and doctors and that, but at the end of the day there are very few that are sort of my age. And if you were put in a children's ward or whatever, then you're with a bunch of kids. So you can't win, you're either with a bunch of older people or you're with a bunch of kids, so you pick the least worst. I can't be doing with kids, they drive me nuts.

(Steven)

It seems that Steven can only conceive of the care setting in terms of 'least worst' which suggests a lack of awareness of the existence of age-specific units and despite saying that he could talk to the doctors and nurses, unlike Michelle, he appears to have found little solace in this opportunity. Clearly he found being treated with the elderly challenging but the prospect of a children's ward was no more appealing, as he graphically said the kids would 'drive him nuts'. At the age of 18, Steven might be expected to find the prospect of being treated on a children's ward unacceptable; however, Ruth at the age of 14 also found such an environment demoralizing. The following extract was written by Ruth, not for the purpose of this research, but because one of the ways she dealt with her experience of cancer was to write in a variety of forms including poetry. She has kindly allowed me to quote from some of her work:

As a 14 year old . . . it is not easy to have to be treated on a children's ward – no matter how caring and understanding the staff may be. While I could appreciate how poorly all the children on the ward were – and that the majority of them were much younger than myself – to have 'lights out' at 8 p.m. somehow added to the humiliation I was feeling and I fully support the need for special units for teenagers who have to be in hospital for long periods as advocated by the Teenage Cancer Trust.

(Ruth)

Interestingly, a survivor of childhood cancer and ex-postgraduate student of mine, Steve, who had been treated as a child of 10 on a children's ward alongside teenagers, offered to contribute a narrative reflecting on what he believed the teenagers were facing on the children's ward where he had been treated more than 10 years earlier:

When I was in hospital, there was a boy who was age 17/18. He kept himself to himself and didn't really mix. You wouldn't want to put a teenager in an adult ward as the age gap would seem too wide, however, he did seem to be out of place in the same ward as small children with pictures of animals on the walls. In my opinion, what is needed is somewhere in between the children's ward and adult ward. Or a defined room/communal space where young adults can be treated like young adults to relax and socialize. Most of the décor, etc. in the children's ward resembled that of a nursery, which is not really appropriate for patients aged 16–18. If I was an adolescent with cancer, I would like to think I would be on a ward with people of a similar age where you can retain some normality. For example, instead of having a room with baby's toys, etc., there could be computers or televisions or a place to listen to music. I suppose mainly just somewhere to sit in the day when you feel a bit lonely and want to take your mind off things and don't want to be surrounded by screaming children. It would be good to have space to sit and talk to people in a similar situation and discuss things if you wanted to. I'm sure you make good friends in this way. I found the worst thing was being stuck in bed all day with very little to do. I was aged 10–11 when I was having treatment but I already felt a little 'old' for sitting in the play room and so I did tend to stay in bed a lot. There was no type of similar room for slightly older children or adolescents . . . this would definitely have been a good thing. There were also less activities for the older ones, all they could do was read or watch TV, whereas the younger ones had games and education tutors, etc. that weren't aimed at older ones.

(Steve)

This reflection was unprompted by me and is indicative that, based on the memories of his childhood experience subsequently mediated by time and some maturity; he has identified the same issues as Ruth.

Philip's account of being treated alongside older patients mirrors that of Steven, yet he felt so ill that he questions whether being in a more appropriate environment would actually have made much difference:

Yeah, I'd say the next youngest person was probably in his fifties, so it was a bit bizarre, that was one of the reasons why they put me in my own room, I was lucky there was one available so they put me in there knowing that I was younger and that and I was getting a lot of visitors and things so that was alright. To be honest with you, I had a bit of a rough time in hospital with pain, they couldn't take the pain away so a lot of the time I was nodding off and people were there but

> I wasn't really with it. I was off my face on drugs and things so I didn't really know what was going on so if I had been on a younger ward, I don't think it would have made much difference anyway.
>
> (Philip)

However, Gemma, who was treated in a general ward with older people around her, was kept largely in isolation to prevent infection and in contrast to Philip, her lack of visitors – particularly over the Christmas period, left her feeling lonely and isolated. Her parents had emigrated to New Zealand and, as we can see, her friends did not visit:

> In a hospital over Christmas, absolutely awful. I didn't like being there because you can't do anything. Very nice room and everything and you've got your own TV and have your own bathroom but just so boring. Just nothing to do all day, and playing patience for probably about four hours a day. There was this chap that used to come in, he was from a chaplaincy, I told him I wasn't a believer but we used to just chat about things. Very few [friends] wanted to come in because they thought they were going to bring germs and everything so they didn't bother come and visiting, which I got really annoyed by. I lost my hair when I was in there so that was quite a low point. I got very angry at Dave [boyfriend] because he never came until late afternoon ... and he's never been one for getting up early and he's very unorganized so it took him ages to get stuff sorted in the morning and then come and see me. But it was just very, very boring and just having more drugs pumped into me and more crap treatment and I was feeling quite down about everything.
>
> (Gemma)

It is tempting to speculate that if Gemma had been on an age-specific unit she might have felt less bored and isolated. However, she said that at 23 she would have felt out of place on a teenage ward, yet at the same time everyone else on the ward she was placed on was very elderly and 'looked very shocked because they don't expect to see someone younger'. The TCT catchment age would in fact have included Gemma at 23, yet her perception was that it would all have been teenagers and she would have felt marginalized, but as we see in the following quote she was sure that there must be others of her age and questioned where they were as she had not encountered any:

> So even when I went for my chemo, there were people who used to look twice at you. It was like 'Why are you here?' When I go for my check-ups now, I think they think I'm actually waiting for someone. A few people have asked if my friend has gone in yet. I was, like,

'Well, it's actually me that's going in.' It was quite strange, I have not ever seen anybody yet on my treatments, or even my check-ups that's actually my age. So I don't know where they're all going because I'm sure there must be a few.

(Gemma)

Someone who would have been near to Gemma in age was Kelly. However, she was not admitted as an inpatient, instead receiving her chemotherapy as a day patient at a cancer unit. At 26, Kelly was the oldest participant, and had experience of working with the elderly. Despite the combination of these factors suggesting that being treated alongside them might have been less challenging, like Gemma, she had encountered no other patients in her age group and this was a source of some concern to her:

I remember when I first went to the cancer unit, I was sat there and it sounds awful, but I was looking around and everyone looked so old. And I could see them looking at me as if to say, 'Oh, gosh, she's young.' And I was, like, 'Oh', and even when I go in for treatments, [there's] never anyone my [age] ... they're all quite a bit older than me ... and I was ... a bit self-conscious really. You know, because you could definitely see them all looking, because it's just that sort of room. I mean, everyone's nice, but you sort of see them going 'Oh, look, what's she doing here?' I mean, I've got used to it now but yes, they're definitely all a lot, a lot older. I mean, most of them are like retired and ... you think 'Oh God ...' I know you shouldn't think like that. You think, 'Oh, is there nobody just like me?' ... you know, you can feel a bit intimidated really. So, it'd be nice to have a chat with somebody my age, see how they cope, if they've got kids as well or with their jobs, you know, how they've managed.

(Kelly)

So despite the 'advantages' of Kelly's slightly older age, her greater level of independence and maturity, she still experienced feelings of isolation, believing that she was the only young mother to be undergoing such an illness and treatment. The stresses of being treated on an inappropriate ward were reflected on by Deborah, a staff nurse on the TCT ward:

People who had been on adult wards at times said that it was depressing and miserable to be surrounded by old people dying ... One of the girls I spoke to the other week had been on a kiddies' oncology ward for brain surgery, she was very much aware of her lack of dignity and privacy. And everything seemed to be focused for kids there. The theme of the [TCT] ward isn't the same because the focus on here is for the teenagers. So, say, on other wards you generally tend to find that the way the ward's run, they're going to have to pretty much fit in with, whereas down here the focus is the other way round.

(Deborah)

However, Ross at 23 had chosen to be situated on an adult ward in preference to the TCT ward. Ross had opted for a package that, for him, offered the best of both worlds. At the time of his diagnosis he was running his own business and living with his partner Hannah and felt he would have less in common with the younger teenagers than with the older patients on the adult ward. Despite the fact that Ross had chosen to stay on the adult ward, most of his treatment took place on the specialist ward and he said the following about his setting of care:

They said I could be treated here [TCT ward] or upstairs [adult ward] ... I've shared wards with people my own age or very similar, you know, up to old people. Well, I get on well with all ages, you know, so I don't mind ... like, I was with one chap and he'd be in his fifties and he was a farmer and me and him were chatting for hours about agricultural things you know ... Yes, but usually when I've been having treatment ... I don't feel too brill, so I don't feel like coming down ... I'm usually quite happy just sat upstairs.

(Ross)

Yet what Ross did acknowledge was that while he felt he could make a better connection with the patients on the adult ward, the opposite was the case with the staff with whom he had a more satisfactory relationship on the TCT ward. His doctor was based on the TCT ward and Ross said the following about his interactions with the staff:

They look after me down here. You know that's where my doctor's based. And they're excellent ... very caring and if there's anything that's worrying you they'll explain everything, you know, time and time again if that's what you want ... they maybe do spend a bit more time with you.

(Ross)

Ross's experience suggests that at the upper end of the age range the flexibility of combining care settings may be preferable to some young adults. Ross's life stage and experience appear to have resulted in him feeling more at ease with older patients, and like Gemma, he felt that he would have little in common with teenagers. This perspective offers a contrast to some of the accounts we have already heard in this chapter, again demonstrating that as well as being on the cusp of services, the young adults are in a transitional life stage and may thus have different and changing needs.

Lessening isolation – restoring 'normality': drawing comparisons between care settings

The majority of experiences presented thus far suggest that being treated in a non-specialist care setting results in young adults feeling a sense of isolation and disempowerment. The following accounts address a range of experiences, some of which are offered by those who had been treated in both the non-age-specific and the age-specific care settings and were as a result able to draw some comparisons that illuminate further what age-appropriate care might offer.

However, we begin with Dawn, a young woman who had not been treated on the TCT ward, but who had been invited to make visits there. Both she, and others who had had a similar opportunity to visit a specialist unit, said that the knowledge that other young people in their age group were undergoing a similar experience reduced feelings of isolation and the perception that they were the only teenagers to be undergoing treatment for cancer. Cancer had been believed by these young adults to be an illness of the aged and being the only young people among the elderly on adult wards only served to reinforce this misconception and the consequent feeling of being 'different'.

Dawn, who was being treated in a non-specialist ward located in a hospital near to a TCT unit, was encouraged to attend the TCT ward's weekly coffee mornings. She found this immensely helpful and her experience also allowed her to make some comparisons between the settings of care. Of the general ward she had been treated on, she said:

> Quite frightening really because I had no-one to talk to, so that made me more conscious not coming out of my room. But then I got to meet quite a few people because you get talking, don't you, eventually? And I met quite a lot of people but unfortunately most of them, most of them have died.
>
> (Dawn)

In contrast, her visits to the TCT ward elicited the following comment:

> I've met quite a few patients up there and they seem really nice. So, yes, I would have [liked to be treated there] because they do activities and go out and stuff like that. [On the general ward] they won't let

you go out. Games and stuff like that ... would have been quite
interesting really ... perk you up a bit, wouldn't it?

(Dawn)

Offering the opportunity to patients from other wards to use the facilities and
interact with patients on the specialist ward was recognized as important by
Cat, the activities coordinator on the TCT ward:

> We do get people from adult wards ... if they're under 25, we try and
> get them involved and just say you can borrow our facilities, the
> internet or come to our sessions ... they can make a cup of tea or, just
> little things that you don't really think of which we take for granted
> here. But on an adult ward they're just sat in their rooms and they're
> not doing anything and you come down here and they've all got
> activities to do. They've got all the facilities, whatever they want ... if
> they were just on an adult ward, they wouldn't be mixing with their
> own peers, they would be with old people or middle-aged people and
> not really in the right age group ... here they are mixing with their
> peers and they are doing activities that they would do at school and
> doing like media studies and we do lots of different accreditations for
> them as well and things like that ... stuck on an adult ward, not
> mixing, they would lose a lot of social skills ... here they help each
> other, talk about different experiences ... they would be talking
> about 'What have you got?' and 'How long have you been here?' and
> just making friends and just sharing, because you're not on your own
> and you're not the only one.

(Cat)

Adrian had been treated on both a specialist ward for young adults and a
general ward, thus he was able to draw an informed comparison. The account
of his stay on the specialist ward suggests that the advantages of a relaxed
environment where he could make snacks when he felt like it and his girlfriend Cindy was allowed to stay overnight made a significant difference to
the quality of his experience:

> 'If you want anything, just go into the fridge, help yourself, go in the
> kitchen if you want cereal, if you want a brew go make a brew.' It's
> just little things like that, you know. And they used to come round
> and they'd just like throw sweets on your bed and chocolate bars and
> ... Basically, you write down on a bit of paper what you wanted and
> by dinner time it would be there for you. So it's about having the
> choice as well, I think ... [It makes you feel] a bit more independent,
> in control like ... the best moment, I think, it would have been when

> Cindy used to come ... and we'd just sit on a settee like you would at home, obviously I'd have my line in my arm and be having my treatment but I was able to walk about, and we'd just sit and cuddle up and like watch a DVD sort of thing in the DVD room.
>
> (Adrian)

Here we see that the small interactions can change the quality of experience, in Adrian's account the quality of care is not the issue, rather it is the 'atmosphere'. As he said, it is the 'little things' that make a difference and this was enhanced by the opportunity to cuddle up on the sofa with his girlfriend watching DVDs, thus bringing an element of normality into his life. But crucially, Adrian also referred to the significance of independence; this may only be related to relatively minor choices like what to eat or when, but for this age group it appears to be of fundamental importance to maintain vestiges of autonomy in whatever way is possible. This is a theme that will be explored in greater detail in the next chapter.

Cindy's mother, also present for some of the interview, offered her opinion on a contrasting experience. Commenting on the inappropriateness of the general ward, she said the following:

> We complained when he was in there ... they brought his dinner round and it was, I always remember, [in] those little disposable paper dishes you do for kids' parties, you put jelly in and things like that. He had one of those with some soup and another one with about six chips, and it was like 'Are you having a laugh?' you know. They actually said, 'If you want to go and buy something, you're quite welcome to.'
>
> (Cindy's mother)

This contrasts with Michelle's more positive experience of a general ward and suggests that Adrian's life stage was not recognized by staff as significant. So much independence has been lost that to feel institutionalized and that choice has been denied in apparently minor – but crucial – ways only serves to lower morale further. Even the ability to make the choice of helping himself to cereal and make a cup of tea clearly has significance under these circumstances. A relatively minimal level of autonomy signified even in such a prosaic way can have a disproportionately beneficial effect on a young adult who has lost independence, as Adrian said it made him feel 'in control' of at least some aspects of his life.

The account that offers the most compelling evidence about the difference the care setting can make was given by Emma. She had initially been treated on a general ward, but her refusal to continue treatment because of her intense dislike of the care setting had resulted in her eventual referral to a specialist unit where the environment, atmosphere and care were experienced by her as being so much better that she agreed to comply. Of the non-age-specific setting she said:

> I hate it. They're horrible. They don't speak to you, the youngest person's probably about sixty. You're not allowed to take anyone with you. Well, I did take him [my partner] with me but they kept sending him out because they didn't have enough seats because the room's just about this big [indicating a small space]. The second time I took my mum and my sister. Because I don't drive, they took us there but then they wouldn't bring us back. We had to get the bus. They're horrible. [It] just seemed to me they were there because it was their job, not because they cared. They said, 'Oh, if it hurts, tell me it's hurting, we'll put down chemotherapy.' So I told them it's hurting, they just said, 'Oh, well, what do you expect, we can't put it any lower you'll be here all day.' And there was like two staff working with about ten people which I didn't think was a good thing either, they didn't have time. And when I finished, they didn't even say 'Bye' or nothing, [I] just went. They told me I was the youngest person that goes there. If I had to carry on [there], I wasn't going to go for anymore [treatment].
>
> (Emma)

Emma's extreme dislike of the non-specialist setting extended to her belief that the older patients were getting preferential treatment and being offered massage that was not available to her. While her partner Gary disagreed that she was being discriminated against, her negative perception was over-riding. Emma's reaction may or may not have been justified in the sense of her being 'right', nevertheless, if such mis/perceptions are not understood or addressed in the care setting, non-compliance may result.[1] Such was the strength of Emma's resistance to being treated in this environment it is likely that her cancer would have remained untreated had the option of specialist care not been sought out by her Macmillan nurse and agreed to by the consultant and the specialist facility. At the time of the interview Emma had visited the specialist facility once, although it was situated much further away from her home, her willingness to agree to treatment there was heavily influenced by the positive impression made by the staff and the environment:

> They're younger people, they're nicer, you can take people with you and [they] seem to more, like, care about you being ill ... It's better, you have more space, more nice staff. People there are my own age so I can talk to them. I've only been there once. They took me out for a

meal and I can't wait to go back on Thursday. I'm quite looking forward to it.

(Emma)

To have moved from the position of refusing treatment to almost looking forward to it represents a dramatic shift in attitude brought about almost entirely by a difference in approach and culture in a setting that recognized Emma's non-compliance and hostility as at least in part being age-related. The relatively modest act of taking her out for a meal had a huge symbolic significance and transformed her relationship with the staff who were then perceived as treating her primarily as an individual and, second, as a cancer patient. There were also the additional benefits of patients in her own age group to whom she could talk and the fact that her boyfriend could stay with her.

One young woman, Sunita, who had agreed to participate in the research was, on the day of my visit to the specialist ward, too ill to talk to me. However, her mother and sister were visiting at the time and after I had left the room, her sister came out to find me and wanted to tell me about Sunita's experience of care. This issue was raised spontaneously by her as she was not aware of what aspect of the cancer experience interested me. Sunita's sister did not want to be recorded so the following is a summary of my discussion with her based on notes taken immediately after our talk and with her consent.

She told me that when first diagnosed nearly four years previously her sister, Sunita, had been taken to an admissions ward in a general hospital and had subsequently stayed on that ward in a side room for six months. During that period she had not been allowed any home visits – even if her condition might have allowed it – as there was a danger that no bed would be found for her on her return even if she had left only for a weekend. No criticism was made of the medical treatment on the ward, but Sunita's sister was very critical of the lack of recognition that a teenager would find being 'incarcerated' while surrounded by the elderly a profoundly distressing and depressing experience. Her sister spoke of Sunita describing her stay in this room as being 'locked up like a caged animal'. Indeed, during a later conversation a member of the ward staff said that Sunita had been forced to use a commode in the isolation room as it had no en suite facilities, thus she was not even allowed to emerge to use the toilet.

After her six-month stay on this ward Sunita enjoyed a three-year remission from the cancer and during this period went to university. However, she had apparently been so deeply scarred by her stay in hospital under these conditions that she suffered severe emotional and psychological damage. Her sister pointed out that these three years might have been her only opportunity for anything resembling a normal life as a young adult but they had been blighted, not just by concerns over the illness and a possible relapse, but by an ongoing post-traumatic effect from the claustrophobic nature of her time in isolation on the ward. She also said that there had been no follow-up counselling or support or any advice about future fertility problems and that staff on the ward had seemed ill prepared to manage or respond to the anxieties of young adults which may differ significantly from those of older adults.

Since Sunita had been on the TCT ward, despite being gravely ill, she experienced the environment as supportive and appropriate to the age group. Her identity as a young adult was recognized and respected, but her sister said it had come too late, she believed that the quality of Sunita's remaining life had been damaged beyond repair. Her sister also said that at the time Sunita had been on the non-specialist ward the family had thought that she was extremely rare in having cancer at this age and it was only since she had been on the TCT ward that they realized that other young adults had cancer too. This realization had resulted in both Sunita and her family feeling less isolated and 'unusual'. This observation is an echo of others whose attendance at the TCT coffee mornings or ability to visit the ward and utilize its facilities had reduced their sense of isolation, marginalization and 'difference'.

The specialist setting

We have seen a variety of distressing experiences that stem from care on a ward where the regime does not address the age-related needs of young adulthood. Yet Deborah (staff nurse on a TCT ward) suggested that through an understanding of the characteristics of the age group it is possible to organize ward routine in a more age-appropriate way. Though the majority of participants treated on specialist wards had not also experienced a non-specialist care setting, they were nevertheless able to recognize the distinctive and age-appropriate characteristics of the specialist environment. Nicola, treated only on a young oncology unit, said the following about the difference she believed it had made to her quality of experience:

> A hell of a lot of difference ... the majority of us were about 16, 17, so we were all going through the same sort of fears and feelings, and we were able to talk about it ... and I befriended quite a few people there which was lovely, it was really, really nice ... because of me being on the young oncology unit, they treated us as mates ... they didn't treat you as patient/nurse sort of system of 'Get up, get this, do this, do that' ... because they were so in tune with the young people ... they said, 'If you want something to eat, there's the kitchen. It's stocked full of bits and pieces that we know you're able to eat because of your mouth being so sore and things. And if you want a hand or a

chat just give us a, just let us know.' And it was lovely . . . it was like a family almost. And it was so nice that on my birthday they made me a card and they passed it round the whole nurses' station and all the other kids that were in there signed it and everything. It was wonderful, it was really nice, and I got a birthday present as well. Not much, but it was a birthday present.

(Nicola)

Similarly of the (different) specialist ward where she was treated Charlotte said, 'It's alright . . . it's like they're all friendly in there.' She went on to describe the sitting room area with sofas and television as being homely and almost like being in a family. She also mentioned that she had been offered music and art therapy and had discovered a creative ability of which she had previously been unaware.

Having 'something to do' is also likely to raise morale, at an age where boredom is hated as can be seen in Donovan's quote:

It's alright, it's something to do, [there's] a lot of people when I go out on the corridors . . . it's good when there's people milling about . . . so there's something to do . . . I hate it when there's nothing to do. They think about it [activities] a lot more. There's a lot more to do like in day room and they have loads of stuff like computers, they have a lot more priority to do stuff and keep you occupied. Yes, it passes time, makes it quicker, the day goes quicker so it makes it better then because you don't feel like you're in all day.

(Donovan)

So we can see from Donovan's quote that as well as the relaxed atmosphere, the sense of purpose is crucial to mitigate the threat of boredom and of time dragging and this resonates with Dawn's observation that such an environment would 'perk you up'. Ricky too made a point of saying how beneficial such opportunities had been as he had undertaken activities he might not have tried had he not been ill, and though he had not experienced care on an adult ward himself, he commented on what other patients had told him about it:

It's not like any wards in other hospitals where you're just all cooped up in big long lines. It's more like one big family up here . . . I have talked to a few that have been on the adult ward and they just say it's awful. It's doesn't exactly feel like a ward up here though. It feels more like a youth clubby type thing . . . It's good, they've always got activities going off and stuff like that . . . You've got CD player, TV, big comfy beds. Over like a weekend, that's really good. [I've] been to

Lakeside which is like an adventure week-type thing. I've also been on a sailing trip with the Ocean Youth Trust, which was sailing round the south coast. That was good as well. And then they do yearly Alton Tower trips and they do trips to concerts and all sorts like that.

(Ricky)

The references to being like 'a family', the 'youth club' atmosphere and being treated 'like mates' are woven throughout the quotes on the specialist setting and as Donovan said: 'The staff are alright, you can have a laugh with some of them.' Of the same ward, Hoody said the atmosphere and the nurses on the TCT ward helped to 'keep you positive'. He added that the last thing he or the other patients wanted was to be surrounded by staff 'who are like sad and stuff', again emphasizing the importance of emulating some 'normality'. This need is clearly well understood by staff as demonstrated in the following quote from Diane, the sister in a TCT ward:

They look to us to, to create a positive atmosphere ... a very relaxed and optimistic, chatty atmosphere really. And always to keep the humour in the situation as and when appropriate ... even sometimes in what seems to be very low situations, they still turn to us for that. And a lot of them say that's what they miss in the atmosphere, if they go to another ward, really is the general banter, the way we converse with them ... which sometimes is very hard to identify to other units, like adult units and paediatric units ... the ones who seem to have the most issues are the ones who come from the adult wards. They don't feel safe on the adult wards – they are safe and they receive the same care, but what I think they don't get is the conversation, is the fact that somebody knows them, the fact that somebody knows what's going on in their life and what's happening to them. And they don't identify that the staff seem to be aware of that [on the adult ward] ... a lot of it [on the specialist ward] is just the banter and the chat and it does seem to identify to them that we know what's wrong and we know what's going on with them and that we're in control of the situation for them.

(Diane)

Another member of the team in the specialist ward said that the patients loved the friendly banter that could verge on the 'pseudo rude' at times; but that the staff's expertise and in-depth understanding of the young people and their needs meant that they were skilled in the art of entering into this type of dialogue while maintaining a good professional relationship. Deborah, the TCT staff nurse who had also worked on adult oncology wards, made the point that the TCT ward tended to be organized around characteristic 'teen-age' patterns such as sleeping late, so apart from the essential administration of medication, the young people might still be asleep at lunch time as they were not required to fit in to the usual rigidity of ward routine. Diane also used the word 'fun' on several occasions, and qualified her use of the word by admitting that this was an unusual term to apply to such an environment but said that while judging when it was appropriate, she would have 'a laugh and a joke' with the patients and that this made the ward a much more acceptable place for them to be.

Simon, a learning mentor on the TCT ward, recognized the social and emotional needs of the young people, particularly in terms of isolation and the potential loss of autonomy and identity. His comment reflects the same approach adopted by Diane and Deborah:

> ... visiting hours are all day, every day and parents stay here and patients can get up when they want to, go to bed when they want to, within reason, as long as they're not disturbing other patients and try and keep it informal and try and keep it reasonably fun, I suppose.
>
> (Simon)

Simon also said that while it was difficult to create 'normality', it could be achieved to some extent through a process of empowering the young people:

> We try and involve teenagers in as much of the decision-making as we can, and not cut them out of the loop at any point. So if there's a discussion, we don't have it with the parents, we have it with them and the parents are there ... I mean things like amputation, they're coached to decide whether to do that or not. And they have a lot of input there ... we try and empower them with the psycho-social side of the unit here.
>
> (Simon)

So we can see that alongside the relaxed 'jokey' environment of the specialist ward representing one kind of 'normality' is the accompanying provision of professional advice and mentoring that serves to empower the young adults and restore some of their lost independence and decision-making powers. The balance here needs to be skilfully managed – staff may not only have to recognize needs that are variable from one young person to another, but also changeable from day to day in an individual according to the stage of the illness and their mood and morale.

Sustaining old friendships – making new friendships

From the material presented thus far, it seems clear that the specialist care setting is experienced as positive. However, given the limited number of specialist wards that exist in the UK, those who are treated in one that is far from home may feel isolated from friends and family, indeed, proximity to home was an issue for some. Yet, while being near to home meant that in theory friends could visit, some participants said that not only did they feel too ill to make the effort to have visitors other than close family; they did not want their friends to see them in such circumstances:

> [We're] really good friends and he [Tom] phones me up once every two days ... he says, 'Look, Nathan, I can't bloody phone you up all the time because I've got like me dad "That phone bill's going up and up"' ... I'm off on holiday with Tom soon ... and, yes, I just can't wait for things to happen like that ... he's really my best friend but I don't want him to visit me because I got, like, no hair and pale and stuff like that. And I don't like him to see me like this.
>
> (Nathan)

Nathan lived close to the TCT ward and had received all his treatment there, he praised the staff and valued the environment of care, yet despite the fact that his friends lived close enough to visit, he did not want his future relationships with them to be affected by having seen him in what he perceived as an unacceptable state.

In contrast, we remember that in Gemma's case it was her friends who were reluctant to visit rather than any resistance on her part, and this left her lonely and isolated on a general ward. Similarly, Donovan whose friends lived near to the specialist ward on which he was treated said: 'Friends don't really come in, they don't really know what to say ... It's just like, it's hard, you don't know what to say, do you ... they just don't bother'.

Discussions with staff on the specialist wards indicated that visitors are regarded as important and it was clear that friends are encouraged not only to visit but also to participate in the activities organized for the patients. However, staff were also aware that friends could feel intimidated by the prospect of visiting the ward and needed reassurance that they would be welcomed. The concern is that if the patients lose touch with friends, then the return to school, college or work can be much harder, thus every effort is made to maximize the maintenance of friendships to help with later reintegration during recovery. However, at this stage in life there may be factors that constrain friends from visiting. Chapter 5 considers the fact that friends are moving on while the young cancer patient's life appears to be at a standstill, thus suggesting that any encouragement to both the patients and their friends that will help to sustain the contact is likely to prove beneficial in the longer term.

In contrast to Nathan's resistance to his friends visiting, Hoody had welcomed those who did and in comparison to Gemma's experience, they had visited in large numbers – again demonstrating the range of experiences. Hoody showed me a photograph album that contained pictures of his friends with him on the specialist ward where they had been welcomed by staff. From the photographs of the groups of teenagers clustered around his bed, it seemed that something akin to a party atmosphere had been achieved in Hoody's small side room. As he told me, a group of ten would visit most weeks, and between visits he could keep in touch through the e-mail contact provided on the ward. However, Hoody also said that he had made close friends with other patients and had been able to reassure a younger patient who also had osteosarcoma in the knee about the surgical procedure he had yet to face.

For most patients, the majority of the time, there was a welcome reduction of feelings of isolation resulting from being on a ward with their peers. Peer support and the knowledge that they were not the only young adults with cancer sustained many of the participants and the value of this aspect of specialist care is well articulated by Hoody:

> Well, in here you don't really notice it but when you get out into the real world, so to speak, and start to see other people, you really do see yourself as being disabled and you know you are really far behind, and that's the good thing about being in here because you're all in the same boat. And you know no-one's better than the other person, you're all doing the same.
>
> (Hoody)

This was reflected on by Diane, the TCT ward sister, who nevertheless acknowledged that there may be occasions when the patients do not want to interact:

> They all have an understanding that they're all at a similar level ... [but] there can be times when on a unit they're not very close and they don't attempt to make friends and join in together. And then there are times when you have a whole group of patients who really gain a lot of social support from being around each other. But I think the knowledge that everyone's in the same boat as them does seem to help them deal with the situation a little better ... the comments that you sometimes get from the girls that they don't need to have the wig on when they're in the ward because everyone else is in the same situation.
>
> (Diane)

Chapter 6 considers the importance of appearance in greater detail, but we have already seen that friends could be discouraged from visiting because of distress over the effects of the illness and treatment on their appearance, thus it seems significant that the ward is a place where peers can be allowed to see the physical manifestations of each other's illnesses without feeling embarrassment.

Simon, the learning mentor on the TCT ward, observed that very close friendships could sometimes be struck up and that these were immensely beneficial for the young people. However, he said that it could then be problematic if one of the friends was discharged, leaving the other on the ward as it was likely that, even if a close bond had been formed, the discharged patient would not visit. Once discharged, there was a reluctance to return unless it was necessitated by further treatment. Nevertheless, Ricky commented on the number of friends he had made on the ward over the years, and Charlotte, who had made a few good friends on the specialist ward, said of one of them:

> Yes, I have [her] phone number and we text a lot and that because she was diagnosed with it after me and she found it quite hard to deal with, whereas I just was happy that they'd found out what it was. So I, like, support her and that and tell her what's going to happen [for] reassurance. That's nice because you're chatting [with] ... people that were going through the same thing. Because, like, you've got your family and that but they don't know what it's like really ... but as someone who's going through it as well that you can talk to.
>
> (Charlotte)

Despite the benefits experienced by the patients in the specialist environment, it was not the preferred place of care for all patients. We have already seen that Ross at the upper end of the age range preferred adult company, but Thomas, at the younger end of the spectrum, at the time of the interview was being treated on the children's ward adjacent to but separate from the TCT ward. He had also been treated on the TCT ward, thus he had experienced both environments. It would have been easy to assume that being surrounded by children would have been annoying for him, but he said the following:

> It doesn't really bother me because I actually prefer it down here to on the teenage ward because it is quite loud sometimes up there. So I prefer a bit of peace and quiet down here, it's nice and quiet sometimes. [On the TCT ward] the TV's on all the time and stuff like that. Yeah, I prefer it down here, a bit quieter. Sometimes it's a bit noisy, no, it's alright, they're [the children] usually quietest. Yes, it's nice down here.
>
> (Thomas)

Such a comment reminds us that although the majority of teenagers and young adults may prefer the specialist and 'age-appropriate' environment, there may also be times of vulnerability when, particularly at the younger end of the age range, the young person does not feel up to the more adolescent activities of a teenage ward and reverts to childhood dependency. However, I was told of only one other case where a patient at the younger end of the spectrum had asked to be moved to a children's ward. Diane, TCT ward sister, said:

> It hasn't come across as a problem on a very regular basis ... there was one particular girl who didn't want to be [with] 17- and 18-year-old patients, she was 13 ... she had regressed quite a lot and wanted to be in an area that was more identifiable with children.
>
> (Diane)

While regression may be characteristic at vulnerable points during the illness for many of the young adults (Self 2005; Zebrack 2006), in the majority of cases it seemed that this could be accommodated within the specialist environment by staff skilled at recognizing the changing needs of the patients.

The impact of the death of a fellow patient

> It is very hard, too, to see other children suffering – and to know many who have not survived the battle (I will never forget the bravery of children like Olivia, Heather, Isabella, Rebecca, Amy, Belinda ... – and their laughter and smiles in the midst of indescribable suffering). Death is not something which many teenagers think about and to be faced with a life-threatening illness and to witness the deaths of other young people whom one has got to know quite well is very hard to come to terms with.
>
> (Ruth)

This extract from Ruth's account speaks powerfully of the impact of the death of a fellow patient – particularly a young patient. One research visit I made to the TCT ward was on the day after a young male patient had died unexpectedly. Thus the mood on the ward was low among both the staff and his fellow patients. I was told by the staff that all the patients had been upset by it, yet no participant mentioned the death. The loss of peers may result not only in an acute sense of loss where friendships have been made, but may also make the young people fear for their own survival. Nicola spoke movingly of the death of a patient who had become her friend:

Unfortunately one of my closer friends died shortly after I'd left [the ward] . . . she had loads and loads of treatment and loads and loads of operations and it just wasn't working for her. So that was a great shock to hear that but . . . [I was] honoured to have met her. And to see her fight the amount that she did fight, but I was pleased that she didn't have to go through it again. Because she'd been through it for quite a few years, and she was getting tired. So it was her way of saying, 'I've given up, I've done my best, I've fought for as long as I have done and I'm not getting anywhere with it so I'm going to give up.' So it was relief in a way but then obviously you're upset because you've lost somebody of your own age . . . The idea of losing somebody that age . . . it's very tragic, it's not what's supposed to happen. They're supposed to be sixty something or seventy something.

(Nicola)

Resonant with Nicola's assumption of it being less of a shock for an older person to die was a comment from Dawn. Dawn, who had not been treated on the TCT ward, said that older people on the ward where she had been treated had died but contrasted their age with hers and said; 'You think, "Oh, am I going to die?" But you've got to think – well, I'm younger.' Nevertheless, although slightly older than her, there had been another patient closer in age than those perceived as 'elderly' who had also died. Dawn was one of the few participants to speak of the death of a fellow and relatively youthful patient and was clearly upset by his loss: 'I mean, there were a couple of young ones like in their thirties and thirty-five . . . who have died. I got really friendly with someone called John and he passed away.' So it seems that the likelihood of the death of a peer, or at least a person relatively close in age is not confined to a specialist ward, and that such losses are likely whatever the setting of care and that, when experienced, they have a profound impact. While no one on the TCT ward mentioned the possible loss of a fellow patient in the same age group, Thomas, on the children's ward, did reflect on the friends he had made on the ward and his hopes that they would keep in touch. However, he also alluded to the possibility that some would not survive:

If I didn't know anybody, it would be a bit daunting really coming in . . . you soon make friends though as . . . at the end of the day we're all here for the same sort of reason, we've all got this damn thing and we want to get rid of it . . . sometimes it can make you a bit upset seeing people . . . who catch it a bit late or who are struggling to get through it but at the end of the day you've just got to concentrate on getting through it yourself.

(Thomas)

Thomas was very positive about his own prospects for recovery and survival, and told me that he believed his cancer had been caught early enough for him to be able to expect a good outcome, yet he was clearly affected by the knowledge that not all of his fellow patients would be as fortunate. Geehan, diagnosed with osteosarcoma at 17, wrote an account of the advantages and disadvantages of being a patient on a TCT unit: 'Perhaps the only real drawback is losing the close friends we make on the ward to this disease and, personally, this is what has proved to be the hardest to deal with' (Geehan 2003: 2682).

Death and bereavement in this age group can have far-reaching effects. A report by the Joseph Rowntree Foundation (Ribbens McCarthy 2005: 2) suggests that the psychological aspects of bereavement pose particular difficulties in relation to the 'normal' development of adolescence and the sociological effects may result in specific vulnerabilities in the context of the relatively powerless and institutional phase of 'youth'. When we add the young person's increased vulnerability and increased feelings of powerlessness due to their illness along with the fear for their own survival, it is clear that the death of a fellow patient is likely to be traumatic even though it is not the death of a family member or necessarily a close friend.

I asked Simon (the learning mentor on the TCT ward) what his experience was of the impact of a death on the ward and he said the following:

> I think that it can be quite a profound effect, yes ... it's not happened a huge amount since I've been here ... patients who pass away while on the ward is quite a rare thing ... patients tend to be on the ward and then treatment will not be working and then it'll be a slower supportive process at home or out in the community somewhere. So I think in that situation only the patients who keep in contact with each other outside the hospital will really be affected ... but things like the guy who died a few days ago, that does have more of an impact because that's so quick.
>
> (Simon)

So, while the impact of the death of a peer can have a profound and shocking effect, it is a relatively rare occurrence on the ward. This helps to put the prospect into perspective and suggests that the benefits of the specialist care setting far outweigh the risk of losing a friend through death. Indeed, it appears from the following quote that deaths are more likely to occur on general wards and this can be just as distressing:

> We went out to visit a chap not so long ago he's 20 ... he was on a ward and the youngest person there was 70 on his ward ... and he said he'll make friends with people and then they'll die, and it was

happening to him quite regularly. And he asked us how many other people his age have this type of cancer, and there was quite a few, and in proportion to the amount of people there are his age and he was amazed because he was the only person they'd had at this hospital with this cancer of that age for, like, the last seven years or something, he was the only one.

(Simon)

In addition to the impact of the deaths of fellow patients, again we see confirmation of the isolation that can be felt by young people who are 'stranded' on a ward with much older patients, who as a consequence believe that they are the only ones of their age with cancer.

Discussion

The need for 'respect' as a basis for following medical advice and compliance with treatment has been established as significant in the wider population, particularly among those groups who may feel that they are disrespected because of their ethnicity or lack of educational attainment (Blanchard and Lurie 2004). Many of the same issues apply to the young adults whose need to be respected for their individuality is fundamental, yet, as we have seen, staff in the non-specialist setting may find it difficult to relate to them. The evidence from the young adults supports Albritton and Bleyer's (2003) assertion with which this chapter began, that the two settings of non-specialist care – adult and paediatric – may not know how to treat young adults.

The young people who had been treated in non-specialist settings of care reacted to their environments in differing ways. Some felt isolated and wanted visitors while others had felt too ill to care. Some found their fellow patients challenging while others found them distracting or good company. Some experienced the staff as uncaring while others found them to have been supportive and understanding. Some liked the privacy of a single room, others felt scared and isolated.

While those in the non-specialist care setting had a wide range of experiences – both positive and negative – those treated in the specialist environment had much more commonality of experience. Many of the extracts taken from accounts of those who have been treated in the specialist environment speak of a culture on the ward that is qualitatively different from the non-specialist setting of care. It is evidenced, for example, by the lack of rigidity in ward routines that acknowledges teenaged preferences, as Thomas et al. (2006: 303) say, 'adherence to treatment regimes can be challenging, especially if it results in loss of autonomy'. But interestingly, it seems that it was those who had experience of both the specialist and the non-specialist setting, and who were as a result able to make a direct comparison, who were most critical of the non-specialist care and most appreciative of the age-specific unit.

The creation of a certain 'atmosphere' in the specialist units was commented on by Diane (TCT ward sister) and this was echoed throughout the testimonies of the young people. It is clear that while many of the young people spoke of the ward as being like a family and referred to staff as being like 'mates' having a laugh and a joke, this interaction was carefully managed by the staff whose central relationship to the young people was as their health care providers, thus necessitating the maintenance of a professional relationship that inspired confidence in their treatment. The maintenance of appropriate boundaries is of fundamental importance, while the banter and jokey atmosphere work well by providing a relaxed environment, at a deeper level, all are aware of the professionalism of the staff and the centrality of their medical skill. Flaherty (2006) quotes Sheets, who warns of the danger of becoming a friend rather than being a professional and as Arbuckle et al. say: 'Expressing empathy while maintaining boundaries and an ability to reflect and develop a flexible approach when working with young people are all very important issues for training' (2005: 239).

Additionally, professional boundaries need to be kept in place because as Morgan and Hubber say, the situation needs to be managed in such a way that dependence does not become an issue. As they point out, while professionals are a small and admittedly important part of the lives of the patients, they are not integral to them (Morgan and Hubber 2004: 134). In a similar vein, Woodgate (2006) reports that the negative side of developing a very close relationship with a member of staff could be that some adolescents have a hard time dealing with a reduction in attention as their health improves. The result can be a feeling of sadness that they are no longer the most 'important' patient and that staff no longer care for them in the same way.

Interestingly Morgan and Hubber report that when the TCT unit in Leeds was set up, the teenagers were asked if the staff should wear uniforms or everyday clothes. Given the value placed on informality and being treated like a 'mate' it is at first sight perhaps surprising that Morgan and Hubber (2004: 134) report this response 'Definitely uniforms, you are professionals, not our friends'; but fundamentally the young people need to have confidence in the staff and a uniform is a signifier of professional expertise that does not preclude the ability to relate to the young people on an individual and age-appropriate level.

My observations on the TCT ward suggest that the environment allowed as normal an engagement as possible with peers undergoing similar experiences. When feeling well enough, the young people would congregate in the day room and did not appear to focus primarily on their illness or treatment but talked about all the usual interests of the age group. Facilities for playing music, computer games, and other such age-appropriate activities made for a relaxed and informal 'youth club' type environment where staff were talked to as friends. Despite this 'youth club' atmosphere, there did not appear to be the usual peer pressure in relationship to self-presentation. Indeed, the ward was a place where the young people felt confident enough to be seen without wigs and make-up by fellow patients. Nevertheless, such an environment may not suit younger teenagers who like Thomas can feel it is too noisy and would rather be on a children's ward, at least during certain periods of their illness and treatment, and Ross, who, at the upper end of the age range, preferred to stay on the adult ward but receive much of his care on the TCT ward, thus indicating a variety of needs in the age band and a need for a fluidity and flexibility that can accommodate changing needs along the continuum.

Despite the variations, I would argue that the diversity represented in this chapter is of less significance than the life stage features that unite the group. For example, as we have seen, being treated with young children or the elderly can be experienced as stressful and exacerbate feelings of isolation. This isolation has been mitigated in cases where young adults have been invited to visit the specialist ward, giving them the opportunity to meet others in the same age group who are also being treated for cancer. Where the young people feel that staff cannot relate to them or their age-specific needs, there are indications that this can compromise compliance as we saw in Emma's case.

The loss of the 'normality' of teenage life that separates young people from their peers, may result in low self-esteem and a belief that they are different in some fundamental way that cannot be compensated for. This can spill over into a reluctance to allow even good friends to visit, as we saw in Nathan's case. If such feelings are experienced while on a non-specialist ward away from the proximity of peers, however good the medical care, the feeling that life is passing by while the young adults are losing touch with youth culture can be acute.

While the experience of being treated with patients of a similar age and at a similar stage of life appears to be preferable for many of the young people, who need to know that they are not the only ones in their age group to have cancer, the potential to make a friend who subsequently dies is a real issue. As Nicola said, young people do not expect their friends to die, and if the death is from an illness that they also have, their own potential mortality becomes conceivable. Nevertheless, the positivity of the experience in general out-weighs the negative impact of such a rare occurrence.

So, it can be seen that specialist centres of care are experienced pre-dominantly as supportive and age-appropriate, yet it is unrealistic to suppose that resources can be found to treat all young adults on wards similar to those offered by the Teenage Cancer Trust facilities. Whelan (2005) says it is im-portant to know how to support young adults who are treated outside the centres of specialist care. The TCT wards clearly offer a model of good practice, while some accounts of treatment on general wards suggest elements of bad or at least insensitive practice. We have seen that while the medical care outside the specialist setting has not come under criticism, the young adults did not always feel 'safe' on non-specialist wards. This was identified by Diane (TCT ward sister) as an issue, even though – as she said – they were of course safe.

Despite the negative experiences, there were nevertheless enough examples of good practice outside the specialist facilities to suggest that an age-appropriate approach can be implemented in a variety of care settings. For example, Michelle's account of her stay on a general ward should be encouraging to both staff and patients in non-specialist environments of care. If life stage issues are understood, the model of the specialist ward and its philosophy of care can be adopted in the non-specialist environment and result in a culture that can transform a setting that may be considered less than ideal.

This chapter has shown that age-appropriate care is of great significance to young adults, but that there are also a variety of needs within the age band to be recognized and catered for. At the present time this seems most likely to be experienced in the specialist environment, but evidence that good practice can be found outside the age-specific wards suggests that models of age-appropriate care could be implemented elsewhere if outreach programmes and the training of staff were undertaken by those with specialist experience who understand so well the particular problems faced by the young adults. This is an issue that is further explored in the final chapter.

Note

1   I am aware that the term 'compliance' carries with it overtones of a power relationship and the concept of obedience. A more appropriate descriptor may be 'therapeutic convergence' as it implies a collaborative relationship between patients and those involved in their care. However, because 'compliance' is more familiar, I shall use it throughout the text while mindful of the aim of achieving something closer to convergence as a goal.

Key points

Through an in depth understanding of the age-related issues, staff in specialist settings can help to do the following:

- reduce isolation and 'difference';
- maintain peer contact;
- offer educational opportunities and activities;
- offer practical help for altered appearance;
- provide an informal, relaxed atmosphere;
- organize ward routine round teenage patterns;
- relieve boredom;
- engage at an age-appropriate level but maintain professional boundaries;
- improve compliance.

A limited awareness of age-related issues in non-specialist settings can result in the care setting being experienced as:

- inappropriate and distressing;
- scary;
- unsupportive;
- isolating;
- intimidating;
- detrimental to compliance;
- lacking privacy and dignity.

However, if the philosophy of age-appropriate care is adopted they can be experienced as supportive.

Flexibility in the care setting may be necessary:

- for those at the younger end of the age range;
- for those at the upper end of the age range;
- at times of vulnerability.

The death of fellow patients:

- is distressing – particularly if in same age group;
- but rare on a specialist unit;
- may be more common in non-specialist setting.

4 Loss of independence

The previous two chapters have focused on topics addressed directly by the NICE Guidance (2005a) and have presented findings which can contribute to the development of policy relating to the provision of age-appropriate services. This chapter and the three that follow are related to more personal issues and themes raised by the participants. They are just as relevant to the patients in terms of age-appropriate care, but are orientated around the individuals' sense of self and well-being. While these issues are of central importance to the young people, their direct relevance to care may not at first sight be so obvious – particularly to those not in the specialist care setting. However, in this chapter and those that follow, I attempt to establish a link between these life-stage-related issues and the setting of care.

This chapter takes as its theme the impact of the illness on the newly found independence that is characteristic of the transition from childhood to adulthood. The struggle for independence is central to this stage of life (Reres 1980). However, whatever independence has been achieved is fragile and likely to be unsustainable when under the kind of stress imposed by a life-threatening illness (Apter 2001; Grinyer 2002a). Crawshaw (2006) says that a cancer diagnosis at this age heightens a young person's dependency and can reverse the trend which is to spend more time away from the family home and with peers. Similarly, Craig points out malignant disease in adolescence comes at a time of increasing independence and she continues by saying that the consequent 'psychological impact of impaired, lost or potentially unachievable independence can be immense ... particularly when the young person sees healthy peers and siblings becoming increasingly independent' (2006: 109).

According to Thornes (2001), illness in adolescence is experienced as particularly threatening and is not well tolerated and Self (2005) says the regression that is a normal response to any major illness can result in resentment and anger when experienced at this life stage when separation from family and the taking on of personal responsibility are the norm. Parents may become over-protective of sons and daughters whose physical limitations throw the whole family back into an earlier dynamic (Hinds et al. 1992; Grinyer 2002a). The effect of feeling independence slipping away is well articulated in the following extract from Ruth's writing:

Perhaps what is hardest – or even impossible – to put into words, however, is the huge psychological impact which the past twelve months have had on me. I am sure that no one ever really thinks that cancer is going to be a reality in their lives – and it is certainly not what one expects as a teenager. For months I felt as if my life was being taken away from me and all I wanted was to 'be normal' again. In the early weeks in hospital, I had to get used to a complete loss of privacy – not only was every part of my body under scrutiny but I was also so weak that I needed help with even the most basic washing and feeding. At a time in adolescence when one is acutely aware of one's body, it was very upsetting to have to be totally reliant on my parents and the nurses for even the most basic washing, toileting and feeding – and without much privacy!

(Ruth)

The extract from Ruth's journal is a powerful account of not only the shock of having cancer at this age, but of the loss of independence and privacy, so newly won during adolescence, and so hard to give up through the illness and its treatment. This was experienced by Ruth, even at 14 at the younger end of the age range when true independence is still unlikely to have been achieved. As Enskar et al. (1997) say, for a teenager to become dependent on parents causes embarrassment and distress, yet for many young people in this age group a return to the parental home for care is their only option.

Despite the fact that Steven wanted to return to his family home, and to be in his own room where he felt 'comfy and safe', his need to retain his independence within that environment seems to have been problematic. He also indicates that the price he paid for the security was an unwelcome amount of fussing and worrying:

I wanted to be at home with my mum and dad. I was happy to be left at home by myself in my own world, my own room and I was quite happy with that. I wanted to be at home which is probably a bit strange, but it was where I felt comfy. Yes, safe, comfy, it was alright ... that's where I wanted to be ... and there were times when I didn't want to be with friends and I didn't want to be with family. 'Cause believe it or not, people can over-care. People can worry and fuss too much and that can get you down a bit. You know, it's like 'I'm alright, just leave me alone.' Or 'Would you like me to go and get you some tea?' or 'Would you like me to make you this and make you that?' No, I can manage myself, I'm not an invalid, you know, I haven't got two broken arms, so I'm sure I can go make myself a cup of tea or cup of coffee or whatever. But people did treat you like that at times. And you can still do stuff yourself, there's nothing stopping you getting off your backside and cooking your own tea ... that was quite annoying ... people are just trying to help and just trying to be kind and all the rest of it, but just over-did it sometimes ... I never felt like I was being treated as a child, I just felt like I was being treated as though I was somebody who couldn't do anything for himself anymore. Like maybe somebody who's disabled in a wheel-chair, who can't get up a flight of stairs, for instance ... I didn't need that help, I was quite happy to just make it on my own. And there were times when I wanted to go to hospital by myself.

(Steven)

It is interesting that Steven draws the distinction between being treated like a child and being treated as a disabled person unable to do anything for him-self, as it can be difficult for parents not to treat their newly dependent sons and daughters as children by reverting to patterns established in earlier childhood, thus slipping back into an outdated family dynamic (Grinyer 2002a). Steven's retreat into the security of his childhood bedroom was ac-companied by a fierce independence that may at first sight seem at odds with his need for safety. It may have been difficult for his family and for him to reconcile the tensions between his simultaneous need for security and in-dependence. It is also interesting that there were times when he did not want either his family or his friends around him, instead choosing solitude, again presenting a challenge to his family (the issue of maintaining friendships is addressed in greater detail in the next chapter).

While Steven needed the security of the family home at the same time as resisting the type of care his parents wanted to give him, Philip was unwilling to relinquish his independence, despite pressure on him to be cared for in his parents' home. Philip had a place to stay at the Outward Bound centre where he was a trainee instructor and he had a strong support network. His parents had to agree, reluctantly, that he would be 'better off' staying where he was, though we have no means of knowing if they really meant this:

I told Mum on the phone that I'd been to the doctor's and I was a bit concerned, they tried coming up there and then, I said, 'Don't bother, there's nothing wrong with me' ... when they first found out, they knew I wouldn't be working [and] they wanted me to go down there, you know, and then they saw how settled I was up here ... I don't think they'd realized quite how settled I was here before. They saw my friends around me and they agreed that I'd be better off up here. They were happy for me to stay on site. They'd have liked to be a bit more involved but I didn't want fussy parents ... I've always been very independent, I mean, I left home just when I was 16, so I've always been independent but ... I get on with them [there's]

nothing they don't know or anything like that, but I just can't cope
with being at home around them all the time.

(Philip)

However, we can see from the extract below, that even when Philip had
negotiated successfully his stay at the Outward Bound centre he found that
his parents' anxiety, manifested as a continual need for reassurance and
checking on his well-being, was intrusive and irritating:

In terms of family care for me, it was a big problem not getting my
Mum and Dad to smother me … they'd be ringing me three or four
times a day to see if I was alright. I was saying, 'I'll speak to you
tomorrow, don't ring me again', I had to be that blunt with them.
They wanted to do their maternal thing and look after me. I had to
just turn round and say, give us a break you're doing my head in, you
know … it took them a while to realize that they were smothering
me … once they just started treating me how they always had done,
they'd ring me up every couple of days or whatever, say how are you
doing?, we could talk about it then, say if I heard anything new, I'd
ring them up and tell them. But certainly them ringing me three or
four times a day was getting beyond a joke … [they wanted] to come
up and move me out of here and take me home. I wasn't having any
of that … during the operation they felt maybe I didn't think they
were very good parents … my Dad told me he was quite upset and he
didn't sleep for a while wondering had he really been that bad a Dad
because I didn't want his help … he couldn't understand how I could
go through what I was without needing their help … he's always
known I'm independent but he just couldn't see how someone of my
age … could cope on my own. Like I say, when he came up and saw
how I was and realized I wasn't just making it up and trying to put a
brave face on it, I was genuinely alright, he was fine. It was only at
first when I was saying, 'Look, don't ring me', they felt like I didn't
want to speak to them … so I just said to him 'More fool you, you
should have told me and I'd have put you straight', yet because they
didn't want to upset me, give me more things to worry about they
kept it to themselves … the way they supported me best was just
knowing that they were only a phone call away, I didn't need them
there 24/7. I just needed to know that if I did want them, all I had to
do was pick up the phone and they would be there and that they
were willing to drive up at the drop of a hat. I knew that if I needed
them they would be five or six hours away, so to me that was as good
as them being in the same house as me.

(Philip)

Steven and Philip were both old enough to have experienced an element of independence, having left home previously and having been in paid employment. However, at the younger end of the age range, Thomas was still dependent on his parents, financially and in many other ways, yet the loss of what little independence he had achieved was felt acutely:

> [I was] starting to do things on my own and then all of a sudden everybody's helping me again. It's like back to square one all over again ... when I'm alright I can get up and down stairs alright on my crutches and go to the toilet on my own but sometimes I do need help getting in the shower and things like that, so I do find it a bit upsetting because I wish I could be able to do it on my own.
>
> (Thomas)

Here we see an echo of Ruth's comments on privacy. At the age of 15, to need help with showering had clearly been an issue for Thomas and he mentions the fact that he had reached an age where he had started to do things on his own, thus the loss of even the relatively limited independence he had achieved was experienced as difficult.

At 19, Nicola was used to being independent and had already started paid employment when she was diagnosed. At the end of this quote Nicola also reflects on the need to re-establish 'normality' (a theme that is addressed in the next chapter) and says the following about her need to ask her parents for help with basic tasks such as eating:

> It was very difficult because I went away to boarding school at the age of 16. And I became very, very independent and then I came home for work and various other reasons and then became ill. And at first I must admit I did quite like the assistance and the help and the smothering. But then it got to a point where I lost the sensation in the tips of my fingers, I couldn't open bottles of coke or tins or anything like that, or even cut my food up with a knife and fork. It was awful ... and my parents were very good actually because they allowed me to struggle until they either realized that I was getting frustrated, or I asked them for help ... I felt like a baby ... but we made a joke out of it ... they'd watch me struggle and then I'd sort of say, 'Look, can you help me cut my steak up?', and my mum would, would cut it up and say, 'There you go, darling' and she'd say, 'Do you want me to mash it up for you as well?' It would be like 'No, don't be so mean!' So it wasn't too bad because everybody knew and everybody was understanding. And I remember going out for lunch with my partner and his friends and I'd again had steak and couldn't cut it up and I sort of glanced at him in a way that said 'Can you help

me please?', without making too much of an issue. So he cut it all up for me and that was it, nothing was said at the meal at all. And it was nice because it felt normal. It's all the normal things that you like because that's what you need that gets you through the day.

(Nicola)

We can see from the quote that humour was the saving grace of a potentially distressing situation for Nicola. Michelle's family also managed the renewed need for dependence well. Michelle had been a student at a university near her parents' home, thus she had not moved far away even when sharing a house with other students. Of this experience, she says:

I enjoyed it when I lived [in the student house], I mean, it was only [locally] that I lived. So, I mean, I was always back here every Sunday for my Sunday dinner. I did enjoy it but I think I preferred it when I moved back home. I prefer living at home anyway because there was three of us in the [student] house and one of the girls moved out ... and then the other lass ... often went home at the weekends. So it was usually just me in this great big house on my own. So I'd invite all my old friends round which was alright, it was nice but then they leave and you're just your own, in a big empty house.

(Michelle)

Michelle had some ambivalence about being alone and her experience of independent living had not been entirely successful. Certainly there is no trace of the fierce bid for independence articulated by Philip. However, although Michelle clearly enjoyed living at home and might have been doing so even if she had not become ill, she did have some concerns about how she was going to find the confidence to leave:

I see it's going to be hard to leave ... if I ever want to leave home and go out and live on my own, I don't know if I'll be able to ... because I'd just be scared in case something happened to me, and there's no-one else there ... I always said that I'd rather move out with some of my friends first, like you see on TV, all mates living together and stuff. Like that first and then move in on your own. But I don't know because some of my friends are living with their boyfriends already and then one is off enjoying the army ... a few of them are still living at home with parents and stuff but they're all moving on now.

(Michelle)

Coupled with her fear that she might find leaving home difficult is the knowledge that her life has progressed at a slower pace than that of her friends who have moved on – leaving her behind. This issue is addressed in greater detail in Chapter 5.

Under different domestic circumstances, Ross was already living with his partner Hannah at the time of his diagnosis. Although Ross was not under pressure to return home for his parents to care for him, they nevertheless wished to be involved. This understandable need for inclusion resulted in Ross's parents making regular visits to stay. Though their increased presence did not result in a direct loss of independence, there are some similarities with other accounts as the joint account from both Ross and Hannah shows:

> My parents live down south so if we'd have still been at Birmingham for treatment, then we would have lived with them and given up our house. But we got the treatment moved, so then we stayed in our own house which I'm glad about ... I haven't lived with them for over five years so it would have been quite difficult adjusting back to it all and I think with the stress and upset of it all – and Hannah – well, you know my parents well but to live with someone else's parents would be quite difficult, wouldn't it? I think it would put quite a strain between all of us really. My parents as well because my mum finds it all particularly difficult to deal with. You know she gets very emotional about all ... they come up like every three weeks because I've been having treatment every three weeks. So usually I have my treatment and go home and then the next weekend they come up and stay for like a long weekend.
>
> (Ross)

> Yes, well, I sort of look after you most of the time and help you. And then when your mum comes here obviously she wants to look after her son and I just feel a bit ... pushed out.
>
> (Hannah)

> Well, that's why we thought living with them there would have been too much conflict, I think, between it all. Yes, we could have ended up all falling out. Because Hannah's working quite a bit, mum kind of gets involved in the kitchen quite a lot, doesn't she? And sort of like cooks most of the meals when they're up and stuff which in a way is very helpful, isn't it, and it saves you a lot of work but, but then again it's sort of like a bit of a invasion of Hannah's space kind of thing. Because you do take pride in your kitchen don't you?
>
> (Ross)

We can see from this exchange between Ross and Hannah that while they have not become dependent on Ross's parents, they have had to make compromises in order to include them in their lives. While both Ross's mother and Hannah want to care for Ross, it is only because of the goodwill and central concern for Ross's welfare that potential conflicts have been avoided.

Mark and his wife were also living in their own home; he pointed out that he and his wife had bought a house when he was 18, but unlike Ross and Hannah they lived only two hundred yards from Mark's parents. While this meant that Mark's parents had no need to stay, Mark nevertheless said: 'She wanted to pamper me ... she can be a fusspot can mother ... but she was far enough away that I could just escape when I wanted.' However, it was clear that Mark's family was close knit and that even under more normal circumstances they would have had almost daily contact.

The increasing involvement of parents in the lives of their adult sons and daughters may also extend to being accompanied to medical consultations. In Chapter 2 we learned that Steven's mother was not present when he received his diagnosis, yet it was she whom he telephoned immediately afterwards with a request to be with him. However, although he valued his parents' advice and support, it is clear that he intended to make his own decisions:

> I still asked my mum and dad what they thought and, and they agreed with me ... But even if they hadn't, at the end of the day, they realized that it's my decision, it's not down to them. It was like when I had some tests done. I had bone marrow taken and I had it taken out of my hip ... my mum and dad had planned to go on holiday. They had it booked a few months previous and they were going to cancel and it took a lot of persuading to get them to go. Well, my level of persuasion was 'If you don't go, I don't go either. I don't go to the hospital.' So it was, like, 'You will go' ... and it got down to the point where I upset my mum but she needed to go, she needed the time away ... she was phoning me every five bloody minutes. 'Are you alright, have you done this, have you done [that] ...?' You know, mums! 'Cause you need space and they do get a bit overpowering do parents at times ... especially your mother.
>
> (Steven)

Here we are reminded of Philip's mother who had to be asked by him not to ring three or four times a day. Steven was in the ambivalent state of wanting and needing his mother to support him and to explain the terminology and treatment while balancing this with his quest for independence through resisting his mother's manifestations of concern that he experienced as 'overpowering'.

Nicola also wanted her mother to be there; again as a parent with some medical knowledge she felt that her mother would help explain the terminology to her:

I wanted my mum to be there because my mum's parents are doctors, so we do have a medical background ... and there's medical terminology that only medical people can understand, so it was nice to be able to go in feeling that we did know a little bit about it ... my mum would be able to translate it if I wasn't able to take it all in at once ... because it's very difficult when you're sat in a room with a desk and a person in a white coat saying, 'These are the medications that you will be on, this is the regime, la, de, da, de, da, de, da, de da.' For you to take it all in at once, it's very, very difficult, and they expect you to. So it was nice to be able to come out of the room and say, 'So, mum, have I got it right that I do this on this day, this on the other day, and I take all these tablets, and anti-sickness tablets that make you feel sick?' ... As they call your name I stood up, and my mum stood up with me and it was nice to have somebody to hold my hand because I was so scared that I needed that bit of moral support and physical support at times, because the number of times that because of my illness I just couldn't stand up, she was there to pick me up, stand me up.

(Nicola)

We see that Nicola not only needed the moral support – she was scared and wanted her mother there as had Michelle in the last chapter; she also needed her mother's medical understanding and her physical support. Yet in this case there appears to be no indication that she found it intrusive or inappropriate. This may suggest a gender difference in that a young man's resistance to dependence on his mother, such as that manifested by Steven and Philip, may be more likely than in the case of young women like Nicola and Michelle who did not appear to feel so stifled.

Nevertheless, the theory that gender can explain why Steven and Philip rejected their mothers' attendance at consultations is not borne out by Mark's account:

I think I've only ever been to one cancer appointment out of about seventy on my own. My wife mainly [comes with me], my mum's been a couple of times when my wife's had to work but I've only ever been once on my own. I'd rather go with somebody off the street than go on my own. It's just that case, just that one in thousand or one in ten thousand chance of it recurring and being told on that day and being on my own.

(Mark)

While Kelly, at the age of 26 and the oldest of the participants, might have been expected to be more likely to attend her hospital appointment on her own or with her husband, we see from the following quote that her mother wanted to be with her:

> They rang a week early and said, 'Can you come in . . . we've got your results back.' And I never thought anything about it. And I said to my mum, 'I've got my hospital appointment through a week early, can you look after the baby?' She says, 'Oh, no, I think I better come with you.' I was like, 'No, I'll be alright, I'll be fine', you know. So I went on my own and that's when I found out and my mum said, 'I wished I'd come with you, because I knew there was something wrong when they called you a week early.'
>
> (Kelly)

It could have been primarily a pragmatic choice for Kelly to have her mother look after the baby rather than accompany her to the hospital, because Kelly also said that when her husband was away she and her daughter stayed with her mother and father at their house. It may be the case that at 26 with her own home, husband and baby, she did not feel the need to establish her independence in the way that those at the younger end of the age range appear to – their independence being more fragile and newly won than Kelly's. This suggests that at Kelly's slightly older age and with increased maturity, the challenge of conceding that she needed help and support was not experienced as undermining in the way that it was for those at the younger end of the age band whose independence was less secure.

Financial independence

Some of the young people in the study were still at school and though they had needed to relinquish a certain amount of independence and, like Ruth and Thomas, become physically dependent on the help of their parents, they had not yet achieved financial independence. However, the older participants had attained a degree of financial independence before the illness and were faced with the loss of this in addition to other losses of autonomy. Illness is expensive, and many families will incur costs that drain their resources (Baldwin 1985; Beresford 1995; Dobson and Middleton 1998). But for those young people attempting to retain independence at a time when their income may have plummeted and they have few material resources or savings, the burden can be immense, as Mark's account of the costs of travelling to hospital appointments illustrates:

> My boss gave me a little bit of office work to do if I wanted it, it was always optional. But if I went back to work I couldn't claim the

insurance for my mortgage even if I was only getting £10 a week. So really it was pointless me trying to do anything. The system really does work against you ... Didn't have a chance to have any savings ... My biggest bugbear was cost of travelling. Nobody ever told me [about a travel grant]. I did look into something but it just wasn't valid for me at the time. I didn't want to rely on hospital transport, going with strangers. It's quite a hard place to get to, so we went on the train and took a bus and my wife came with me, and it would be a £100 round trip.

(Mark)

Here we see yet another manifestation of the desire to maintain in-dependence – Mark did not want to be ferried around by strangers from a hospital transport service despite the high cost of public transport. Yet such costs are incurred at a point when the young person may be unable to work and is reliant on state benefits, thus the situation can be the source of con-siderable stress. Gemma's account of her ongoing financial problems in-dicates the complexity of the benefits system for this age group:

Back in May although I had finished radiotherapy and things were looking up, I was getting stressed about money. I had finished my sick pay and of all things had to do something I never in my life thought I would be doing – claim benefits. I know I shouldn't have but I felt a fraud claiming benefits even though I had no money coming in. I was struggling financially and if it hadn't been for Dave [my boyfriend], I really don't know what I would have done. The process itself takes a ridiculous amount of time and the personal information they ask for felt so intrusive. I was told I wasn't entitled to incapacity benefit as I hadn't paid enough contributions despite working as a staff nurse and them taking a huge chunk of my pay each month. I suppose it's the downfall of having to claim when you have only just started your career. I could claim income support, which was only £40 a week and eventually after two months got housing benefit. I was distraught; I had no other way of getting any income. If I had been on my own I would have had to find someone to move in with as I wouldn't have afforded my rent. I thankfully had a small amount of money in my bank but that soon ran out. I had to rely heavily on Dave for rent payments as he was living with me at the time; he thankfully was getting a good wage. I haven't relied on anyone for money since I started my training and I hate owing money. I love my independence and the money I earn allows me to keep that, it felt awful to have that taken away from me. A lot of things that I had to get went on my credit card, another thing I hate using unless for emergencies. I have now started to get paid from my job and that first pay cheque was amazing. I have my own money, I can start paying people back and my credit card and the stress of not having money is lifted slightly and I no longer have to claim benefits thankfully. I have a set goal of paying off debts as quick as possible and I think I will set up a savings account just in case. I have always thought that I as a nurse would never be without income from work, but as I have found out you don't know what's around the corner.

(Gemma)

Clearly Gemma's experience was worsened considerably by her struggle with the benefits system and her feelings of humiliation at having to subjugate herself to what she perceived as a demeaning process. Gemma did not have the option of returning to her family home as her parents had emigrated to New Zealand, though her fierce independence may have precluded a return to the family for care as an acceptable option even if they had been in the country.

Philip, who struggled to maintain his independence by staying at the Outward Bound centre where he worked, was faced with a financial situation that could have made the fragile situation between him and his parents more difficult:

I was told to claim for Income Support and Incapacity Benefit and then Housing Benefit as well, but they said I wasn't eligible for Incapacity Benefit so they gave me Income Support and that was about £43.00 per week. Then to top that up, I got my Housing Benefit and that was something like £40 per week. At first £40 sounds a lot but when you've got to make up the shortfall in the rent from that £40, all of a sudden you haven't got much money ... Trying to run a car, although you get all your petrol money back to and from the hospital, you get it back once you've filled the car up, so you've still got to have the money there to fill the car ... Well, at the moment I only earn £60 per week, that's all I've earned since I left college, so I don't earn enough to have to pay tax and National Insurance so all the records show that I've not made many contributions so that's why I'm not entitled to it ... the worst thing was I'd been without work for about 7 or 8 weeks before I got my first bit of money through, well, to go from earning £60 per week to then have that stopped and not get another penny for like 7 or 8 weeks was just a joke. I mean, my parents had to bail me out you know a couple of times ... but even once I was getting it, I kept on getting forms through to make sure I was still eligible for it, as if they thought I was making fraudulent claims and always having to justify why I was getting the benefit and [them] asking why I wasn't working ... when I had my Hickman line in they said, well, other people work with it in. I said [in] the sort of job I do I'm not allowed to (trainee Outward Bound instructor). I ended up having to get a letter from the doctor saying I wasn't allowed to do my job with it in ... It was nothing to do with the health service at all, that was the job centre ... they were absolutely shocking throughout the whole thing ... that was the hardest and that's what caused me all the stress. It wasn't my illness at all, it was constantly having to work just to get peanuts to live on each week ... had I not had to claim benefits, then I could just have carried on as normal. Mum and Dad said ... for the hassle you're getting and the stress it's causing you, we'd rather pay you £50 per week and pay your rent for you and you not claim benefits. We very nearly did that.

(Philip)

The additional stress endured by Philip in his dealings with the benefits system is clear; indeed, it appears that the financial situation caused him more concern than his illness. In another example, Adrian had been trying to maintain his independence and to continue living with his girlfriend Cindy, who was 16 at the time. Cindy's mother contributed financially by taking on six different cleaning jobs as well as her main job to help them pay their mortgage, as she said, 'It was a hard time for everybody.' However, Adrian and Cindy were unable to pay their Council Tax, and though Adrian appealed to the Council Tax office stating that he had not been earning any money as a result of his illness, he said the following about their response:

They wouldn't put it on hold, they wanted their money. They sent me a letter saying they were going to send the bailiffs unless it was paid and then I had to grovel to my boss for about three hundred and fifty quid. I got a summons to court when I had cancer and we explained that I wasn't working and the woman in the council said, 'But what's your reason for not paying the bill?' I [said] 'Can't you not see I'm not well? I'm not working, so we've got no money?' 'But what's the reason for not paying the bill?' That's all she kept saying.

(Adrian)

In the end, Adrian's boss paid the outstanding amount for him and Adrian later paid him back when he could afford it. However, at the time of the interview, Adrian and Cindy were living in Cindy's parents' home as they did not have the resources to live independently, demonstrating that dependence can take forms other than reliance on the physical assistance needed during the worst of the illness, and can have an ongoing effect even after recovery. In this case a couple who had been independent were forced back into financial dependency on parents.

While Ross and Hannah had also encountered financial difficulties, they had managed to maintain their independence but this had entailed the selling of Ross's assets and Hannah having to give up her university course for the year in order to work:

> I'm entitled to sick pay, which is £59 a week, and we live together and so we applied for Housing Benefit as well, and we're entitled £25 a week which is fairly insignificant really. We were allowed some help with Council Tax for a while but they seemed to have stopped that for some reason. They never really gave any reasons, just said that we weren't really allowed ... But since you've [Hannah] stopped university, you're working, you know more than you were doing so that's the only reason why we're managing to get by really because Hannah's had to work. I sold [my] trials bike [and] motor bike that was worth quite a lot of money and a tractor. I sold that ... selling assets to try and keep going through it all, you know, and savings are dwindling.
>
> (Ross)

Mark, entitled to sick pay of '£48 a week, I think it was' had a mortgage at the time of his diagnosis. Although he described the mortgage as not being 'massive', his financial problems were still worrying:

> My wife was working [but] by the time we'd paid the bills ... I had insurances, but the stupid thing about the insurance was that I had to pay my mortgage before the insurance would give me my money back ... fortunately my employer looked after me very well, he gave me money ... [and] my parents helped out, of course they did.
>
> (Mark)

Again we see an employer helping out and also parents upon whom a young married couple would hope not to be dependent. Yet in Mark's case he eventually benefited unexpectedly from a mistake made by the insurance company:

> But then I sort of fell lucky [though] I suppose there's no lucky situation in the situation I was in, but I had something called Critical Illness Cover which I didn't know about and it paid my mortgage off and there'd also been a mess-up with the insurance, and they'd been taking double the premium out for twelve months so they had to pay

out twice. So I had about £20,000 in the bank and I blew it. I didn't want it; it was cancer money ... it was like given to me by somebody that I hated and I really didn't want it. Me and my wife lived very well for twelve months. I had two brand new cars, which you can imagine with cars, that sort of lost all that money.

(Mark)

It is interesting that Mark seems to have regarded this money as 'tainted' and so closely associated with his cancer that it appears he wanted to get rid of it. Despite his married status and responsibilities, that he chose to spend the money on cars could be interpreted as being age-related – perhaps stereo-typical of a young man. Five years after the cancer diagnosis, Mark is the father of two children (see Chapter 7) yet he does not entirely regret the choices he made at the time mainly because he is now earning good money. However, Mark also acknowledged that some of the money had in fact been spent on a new kitchen – so we have the juxtaposition of the stereotypical young man's car fantasy with the responsible married man's new kitchen – perhaps more evidence of the cusp upon which this age group rests.

Many of the cases discussed suggest that the complex financial situation the young people find themselves in relationship to benefit is almost in-evitably problematic, and parents and employers are the ones who step into the breach to prevent disaster while entitlements are sorted out. However, Charlotte's account of the support she was given by the social worker on the specialist ward where she was treated demonstrates that with good informa-tion and advice financial problems can be addressed:

Yes, we have a social worker at [the hospital] ... who helps with money problems and helps fill out your forms that you have to get to claim your money and things like that. I can get a disability [benefit] and income support.

(Charlotte)

Charlotte was planning to buy a car with the benefits she had been awarded but said that without the help from the hospital social worker she would not have known what she was entitled to, as no one else had offered any support or advice. Charlotte's grandmother made the following comment:

For instance, when she was going down for this big operation, we went down on the Tuesday and we booked in at a Travelodge, Charlotte, me, her mother and her little sister for two nights which was £52 a night each, so I paid for one night and Julie [Charlotte's mother] paid for another, thinking she was having her operation on the Wednesday, but you didn't have it 'til the Thursday, did you?

> And then she'd to have an emergency operation on the Monday. And this social worker came to intensive care to see Charlotte and I was there. So just talking in general, I said that we'd come down, booked in this hotel, she said, 'Well, give me the bill and I'll get you the money back.' So I said, 'Well, it's in my name not in our Julie's.' She said, 'Oh, it doesn't matter.' So we gave her it and she got us the money back ... and with petrol costs because it's always down the motorway and they've helped out with that as well, haven't they?

Charlotte's experience contrasts strongly with those who endured struggles with the benefits system. This suggests that in addition to the specialist ward offering a supportive care environment, the expertise of social workers dealing with the particular needs of the age group and the complexity of disentangling their entitlements can be of enormous practical assistance to the patient and their family.

Discussion

It is clear from the young people's accounts that the illness brought with it a loss of independence. The age range of the participants suggests that there might be a wide spectrum of experience and attitudes, yet we find that Ruth, diagnosed at 14, found the prospect of the loss of privacy and the physical reliance on her parents as challenging as those at the older end of the range who were facing the loss of a more established independence from their family. While there are differing scenarios represented, such as that of Michelle who clearly wanted to live at home, through to the contrast of Philip who refused to return for care by his parents, we can still see similarities. Michelle recognized that she did not know how or when she might eventually gain her independence, and Philip still had to deal with what he perceived as 'over-anxious fussing' from a distance in addition to severe financial hardship. Although dealing with the situation in different ways, these are young people struggling with a disrupted life trajectory and the loss of not just independence but of the ability to fulfil the 'normal' expectations of the age group.

There is evidence from the accounts that throughout the age range and variety of life styles, the loss of independence was upsetting. Few young adults at this stage of life are likely to have the material or social resources to sustain them through such an experience. The reluctant need to acknowledge that their newly found independence is so easily lost – particularly at a time when, as Craig (2006) points out, peers are establishing their own independence successfully – generates a great deal of distress. Given that under most circumstances it will be parents to whom the young adult turns for support, there is also the likelihood that there will be a reversion to previous de-pendencies and patterns of behaviour redolent of an earlier family dynamic that will be experienced as inappropriate and challenging by all family members.

We have also seen that a manifestation of independence can be to attend medical consultations alone, believing it inappropriate to be accompanied by a parent – usually the mother (Grinyer 2002a). This can present problems not only for the young adult who may be given bad news that they do not un-derstand fully without the support of a family member, it can also be difficult for professionals who are faced with having to balance judgements about capacity, competence and confidentiality. This theme is explored further in the final chapter.

In addition to the loss of physical independence, the loss of financial independence was an issue for some. At this age when so little in terms of material resources have been amassed, and a minimal contribution to state benefits made, young adults may find themselves struggling not only with the loss of financial independence but also be facing real financial hardship, as we saw in Adrian's case when the bailiffs were threatened.

It is clear that the benefits system was challenging. It was experienced as complex and unsympathetic to the age-related needs and financially pre-carious situation in which many young people find themselves. Officials dealing with claims were perceived to be unhelpful and on occasion hostile, and in the cases of hardship presented here it seems that no social worker or other professional involved in the medical care was readily identifiable to assist the young person. Interestingly, the young adults who raised financial issues as a problem were not treated on a specialist ward, thus it seems likely that the complexity of the benefits system was not well understood by pro-fessionals outside the age-specific care setting, suggesting another advantage of the specialist environment where support staff become expert in the benefits system as it applies to teenagers and young adults.

While not of direct clinical significance to the medical professionals providing care, the loss of independence and concerns over financial issues affect the young people at a profound level, and must therefore impact upon their well-being. The example of the social work support that resulted in financial assistance was experienced by Charlotte and her family as im-mensely helpful and supportive. This suggests that specialist expertise in the age-specific care setting can additionally transform the experience in ways that are not directly related to medical care but which impact upon quality of life in a meaningful way and thus may affect compliance and ultimately outcomes.

Key points

The loss of independence is felt acutely because:

- it is fragile in this age group;

- it is experienced across the age spectrum;

- dependence on parents is perceived as a retrograde step;

- there can be a renewal of infantile dependency;

- family dynamics are disrupted;

- financial resources may be limited;

- access to benefits may be difficult.

Suggested improvements are:

- a key worker in an age-specific setting who may have expertise in entitlements;

- such support may improve compliance.

5 Disruption of the life trajectory: the impact on 'normality', life plans and friendships

Central to the life stage of young adulthood is its transitional nature. This is a period of life when many plans are being made and the foundations for the future are being established, as Lewis says:

> These young people are experiencing a period of life when they are initiating major life tasks, including establishing their personal identity, establishing independence, making occupational choices, and developing philosophical and lifestyle choices.
>
> (2005: 242)

We have already seen in the last chapter that independence is threatened in a way that can be found distressing to some of the young adults, and there were indications that regaining 'normality' is of central importance. Normality may relate to the everyday routine activities that we all take for granted, but in this age group it also has more far-reaching implications. It is a time when crucial exams are being taken and careers are being established. Sexual relationships are being formed and some young people will be planning to marry or have a baby. In addition, the increased independence that comes with the transition from childhood to adulthood manifests in expectations of travel and the social activities that are frequently associated with this time of life. The interruption of this trajectory may also have implications for long-term financial prospects as disrupted schooling and a poor attendance record can limit future employability (Craig 2006: 111).

The role of the peer group is also of central significance in this age group (Thornes 2001), yet a cancer diagnosis will separate the young adults from their peers, can result in social isolation and limit interactions to those with family and health professionals (Nishimoto 1995). At a time of life when peer acceptance and a sense of belonging are important to feelings of self-worth (Grant and Roberts 1998), this can add an additional layer of stress.

So, when life-threatening illness puts plans in jeopardy and disrupts friendships, the effect can be felt more acutely than might be the case at other times of life. Nicola conveys eloquently the frustrations she felt at having had her plans thwarted:

> And everyday life is quite hard so your ideas of going to, I don't know, London for a week, can't be done because you physically can't do it. So you set yourself goals that are achievable ... Silly little goals like going for a walk, be able to walk to the end of your street. If you can get to the end of the street and back again, you get a chocolate. And doing that you set yourself up not to fail ... I was pissed off, I was pissed off. I must admit I was pissed off, I couldn't go down to London, I wanted to go to London ...
>
> (Nicola)

For a young woman in her early twenties to have to acknowledge that walking to the end of her street was as much as she could expect to do, in her words, left her feeling 'pissed off'. The emphasis of her repeating twice that she wanted to go to London, and saying three times that she was 'pissed off' eloquently demonstrate the depth of her despair at the constraints imposed by her illness. Younger than Nicola, Thomas's plans may have been more modest, but his frustration at the physical limitations that prevented him from taking part in the 'normal' social life of a teenage boy is clear:

> I like doing football, especially I'm missing that quite a lot because I can't even walk now. I have to use crutches to go everywhere and sometimes a wheelchair as well, so I really do miss things like that. And stuff like rugby and basketball ... just to go for a walk in the park or something like that, just walk round or walk round town or go somewhere and eventually hopefully to be able to ride my bike again so I can go round with my friends and everything, just get back to normal.
>
> (Thomas)

The limitations imposed by James's ALL resonate with Thomas's frustration and similarly refer to the desire for 'normality':

> At the moment the hospital is like a second home to me, it seems like I am always there. I cannot wait until my treatment eases up a bit and I feel stronger again and can start doing the things that I enjoy most. Because of the side effects of the chemotherapy I cannot always go to places where there is a crowd as I am very susceptible to infection, but as soon as I am fit enough and well enough to do what I want, I

will do as much as I possibly can and enjoy myself, and lead a normal life again.

(James)

Hoody's account of attempting to do Christmas shopping while in a wheel-chair shows how a relatively unambitious, but 'taken for granted' activity can signify the losses that have to be endured:

> I went into a record store and my brother just had to leave me be-cause you can't get around the aisles because they're so thin. You know, it gets quite annoying because I just got fed up. I'd been looking forward to going to York shopping for ages and got there. It was just before Christmas because I was shopping and I just had to sit around all day while my brother went and found stuff that I asked for. You know, it's not exactly the way I like to shop.
>
> (Hoody)

An attempt by Hoody to 'normalize' his life by doing a fairly ordinary thing like Christmas shopping seems only to have served to make him feel even less 'normal' and highlighted his dependency. The same can be said for his at-tendance at the school ball despite the support of his friends:

> I managed the school ball before Christmas which was a huge step. I mean, I couldn't stay all night and I got a bit upset when I couldn't get up and dance and the music's so loud you can't really talk. But I try and do as much as I can and my friends have been a great help.
>
> (Hoody)

The frustrations thus far have been related to relatively modest, albeit highly symbolic activities such as going shopping, travelling to London or walking in the park. However, Gemma had had more ambitious plans which included going to New Zealand with her boyfriend to see her parents and working while out there:

> Up until this point everything had been going very smoothly and my life was sliding into place, with my career going well and my personal relationships. I was planning to travel to New Zealand with Dave in March 2004 to work for 6 months and then to Australia travelling around. My parents had moved to New Zealand in May 2003 and so as well as a working holiday, it was to see them and where they had settled. I also had several courses booked to increase my skills within my current job and be able to mentor students, something which I enjoyed doing while working ... I'd just got an E grade which is one

promotion up, and I was just getting into that role and taking on more responsibility at work, doing team leader and link nurse roles. That had to all stop ... any sort of plans whatsoever just got completely thrown to the side. So, quite depressing really ... I was facing cancer treatment that was going to mess up everything I had planned this year and possibly next. I went through periods of feeling extremely angry and frustrated about it all.

(Gemma)

Here we see that Gemma's plans were related to leisure, family and work, yet all had to be cancelled when she was diagnosed with cancer. Up until her diagnosis, her job had been going well, and this is a time when careers are being established and some will be supported by college courses that are crucial to progression. Thus to take time out for illness can lead not only to financial insecurity as we saw in Chapter 4 but also to fears that it will be difficult to get back on the career path. Steven had been attending college as an apprentice alongside his job, and he indicated that having to take time out for illness had been a problem despite the fact that both the college and his employer were supportive:

I ended up being a heavy goods mechanic and I was in my third year there, so with college that caused a bit of a problem really, trying to work at work, go to college and sort of get through everything, get through the cancer ... that, well, that was a bit of a worry at first. It was like, well, I'm two and a half years in, I've only got half a year to go, like, why now? You know, now is not a good time.

(Steven)

In Steven's words 'now is not a good time' and this portrays with clarity the frustration of young people on the threshold of their adult lives who find that they are halted in their tracks. Steven wanted to get on with his life, yet he was missing out on his training, worried about his job security while also feeling that life was passing him by. As a result he went back to work too early:

After I'd had my treatment, I had a short rest period of like a week, which was my biggest mistake ... I really over-rushed going back to work and I didn't just sort of ease myself back into work. It was like, 'Well, I've finished all my treatment now, I've had a week off, I'm getting bored at home, right I'm back at work full time.' I lasted a week, collapsed at work and the doctor signed me off with exhaustion for three weeks, 'You ain't going anywhere, stay in that bed and take it easy' ... and then after that I eased myself back into work, I did a morning three times a week. Then I did a full day three times a week, and then just built my way up.

(Steven)

Although eventually Steven went back to work by building up his hours, he believed that his career had been adversely affected:

> I went for an interview a couple of years ago now and, I can't prove it but I reckon that I didn't get that job because I'd had cancer. Now I can't prove that but I'd like to be able to and I'm 99 per cent sure, because I made it through the initial interview, through the second interview, no problems, I answered all the questions they had to give to me and not a problem. Knew exactly, I had read book after book ... you had to answer certain questions ... which was a doddle. Yet I never got the job. Now they knew I had cancer, now, as I say, I can't prove nothing, but I think that's one of the reasons I didn't get the job. You know but how do you prove it, you can't?

(Steven)

Regardless of whether Steven is right or wrong about why he did not get the job, it was his firm belief that it was the cancer that had prevented him from being appointed. But in addition to the concerns about his job and training is a profound irritation at 'waiting':

> I've got better things to be doing, you know, really, than sitting in hospitals for days on end ... that's a bit frustrating, wanting to get on and that's as annoying to me as anything is that. That annoys me that I had to wait, you know, I'd done enough waiting, I was sick of waiting ... say, my appointment was ten o'clock, I don't think I ever once had an appointment that was running on time. You know, machine had broken down or somebody else was late which put everybody else late, or whatever. And I used to wait there for hours and hours and hours on end, and I don't like waiting or pacing. Oh God, it used to drive me nuts. And you couldn't go anywhere because you never knew when you were going to be called. So it was, like, sit here and wait ... young people are not generally patient ... my grandfather is 77 and he's the most patient man I know. He can sit and read a paper from cover to cover and not miss a word and do all crosswords and puzzles, but I can't do that ... teenagers especially aren't very patient, we're not the best at it, and you do get annoyed, and at times I've shouted, not being nasty, well, not particularly nasty at the people who have been there, at the hospital. But you say, like, well, come on, what the hell's taking so long, you know. I've got

> places to be, I've got things to do you know, I've got a life to live ...
> waiting's the thing, it's hard work.
>
> (Steven)

The waiting that Steven cannot tolerate applies certainly to the hours spent awaiting hospital appointments, but perhaps more profoundly also to the waiting for life to begin or to resume some semblance of normality. He recognizes that teenagers are not renowned for their patience and imagines that perhaps his grandfather would not feel the same sense of frustration. There is an assumption here – rightly or wrongly – that older people are content to read or do the crossword and might use such devices to occupy the time spent waiting for appointments or during convalescence. The implication also seems to be that his grandfather is not waiting for his life to begin but is instead nearing the end of life when such challenges might be expected and can thus be faced with greater equanimity.

A similar frustration was felt by Donovan who said of his treatment 'It's just waste isn't it, just wasting time.' Donovan acknowledged that the treatment was essential to his recovery and was thus clearly not a 'waste of time' in that sense, but his emphasis on the word 'waste' indicates his feeling that life was moving on without him despite the fact that he was having college work brought into the ward so he could continue his studies.

Philip, a trainee Outward Bound instructor was allowed (unpaid) time from work with the expectation that when he was well enough he would return. Clearly the level of fitness required to resume such a job is higher than for a desk-bound occupation. Though Philip was confident that he would complete his training, he was annoyed that his progress had been put back a year:

> At the start, it was a pain because I thought, well, that's 8 months to a year without work that's going to put me back a year, because I'm still in training for what I do but I'm nearing the end of it, you know, so I should have had a full time fully paid job by now, but as a result I'll have to wait till January/February time before I'm ready. So that was the only frustrating bit and that's the main way it's affected work. It's just put me back that time.
>
> (Philip)

We have seen examples of disrupted trajectories from young people who have been in work or training, but Toni had just been accepted on a university course when she was diagnosed:

> I'd just found out that I'd got into university ... So I thought I'll get some money before I go in September, and then it all came about [the cancer] and it turns out I have to defer for a year ... all my

friends went to university last year and I didn't manage to get in last year. So then I tried again this year and I did get in but unfortunately I've got to wait another year before I can go.

(Toni)

Not only did Toni have to relinquish her university place which she hoped to take up at a future date, she had to witness her friends going away to university. This means that even when she does attend university, her life will be out of synchronicity with her friends' lives and her fellow students will be at least two years her senior, her frustration at this delay was clear. Of course, students who elect to take a 'gap year' will also be out of phase with their school year, but this is their choice and the year that they take out is likely to have been filled with experiences that are the antithesis of cancer treatment.

Hoody knew that all his friends would be in the year above him when he returned to school, he was resigned to this and tried to be positive by saying that he did have some friends in the year below him, so he hoped that would help. However, Hoody had been a promising athlete and was coming to terms with the fact that his sporting activities would be affected detrimentally by his illness:

I did quite a bit of swimming and scuba dived a lot but [I was] mainly an athlete, multi events and discus is my main sport. I was aiming for the Nationals in multi events and discus this year but you know when I got this knee injury, I pulled out of multi events ... I couldn't play any sports ... You know, you watch people playing tennis, because I used to play tennis and squash and badminton and all that ... Mum's always saying, 'Oh, you could've gone to the Olympics', at the World Games a couple of years ago they said, 'Oh, we might see you ... at the Olympic Games' ... but now they want me to try for the Paralympics ... who knows, but I suppose the Paralympics is an option ... if you've got osteosarcoma you've always got to have big operations ... and you won't be able to do so much afterwards which affected me quite badly because I enjoyed my sport ... it was fifty, fifty whether they'd amputate or not ... so, you know if I lost my leg, I didn't know how I'd react.

(Hoody)

Vicky was extremely ill at the time of the interview which as a result had to be cut short as she kept falling asleep. However, during the short time we talked she told me how at 15 she had been diagnosed with leukaemia, and had one day been sitting in her classroom at school with all her friends and the next day hospitalized with a life-threatening illness. This sudden change in her life had come as a 'terrible shock' and it appeared that it had taken her some time to believe in the reality of what was happening to her. She had planned to be an English teacher and was concerned at the amount of school she was missing, although she had been allocated a home tutor for seven hours a week (an amount of time that her mother said was unusually generous), she had never been well enough to have any home tuition. She also told me that she had been looking forward to her sixteenth birthday for some time leading up to it, but her plans for a big celebration had been thwarted by the illness which forced her to remain at home in isolation lest she should pick an infection.

Also at the younger end of the age group, Thomas was missing his friends and he too was concerned at the school work he was missing:

> I do miss school quite a lot because I don't see people as much as I used to now because I'm stuck in here all the time or when I am at home they're at school so I can't see them anyway, so every now and then it is good to see my friends but I really miss school. I wish I could go back, I'd go back any day if I could ... I've got a home tutor who comes round, comes into hospital as well and does 5 hours a week with me which is like just one day at school ... she's a nice teacher so we get on quite well so I'm doing alright with that and, hopefully, I should be OK, but it is quite worrying really because all of a sudden everything's just cut off. You're cut off from school and all your friends and everything, it's really strange.
>
> (Thomas)

While many teenage boys might imagine they would welcome time away from school, Thomas's frustration is clear as is his sense of having been 'cut off' from normal life and he indicates that the loss of the normality of school life has also resulted in separation from his friends. Thomas looks forward to being back at school, but Ricky's attempt to return to school and normal life was unsuccessful and as a result he had been unable to take crucial exams:

> I don't think they [the school] wanted to waste their money on the GCSEs for me because they thought I were going to fail and that, because I haven't, you know, been at school doing any work and that ... I just wanted to get some qualifications under my belt. You know, it'd look good on your CV and stuff like that. Help getting a job and stuff like that. But no they didn't even want to know.
>
> (Ricky)

His mother said the following about his failed attempt at reintegration at school:

He went back to school . . . the Macmillan nurse from here came with us and they went to talk to the school and explained everything about him. He'd lost all his hair obviously so he wanted to wear his hat for school, which the headmistress said it was no problem, he could wear a hat. And he only went back for two days, didn't you? Just everywhere he went, teachers screaming at him all day long, 'Take your hat off boy or, . . .', the way the teachers treated him was disgusting so I pulled him out after two days. We had a home tutor again then, when it was GCSE time and he says, 'I know I haven't been to school' he said, 'but I would like to go and sit my GCSEs . . . just to see what I could do' because he's quite good at maths. So I rang the school and I said 'We know he hasn't been but he would like to come and sit the exams.' They told us 'No.' They just didn't think it was worth it, they said, 'If he sits them and fails, he'll be more upset than what he is now' . . . the school were quite disgusting.

(Ricky's mother)

We can see that Ricky's attempts at both reintegration in school and in trying to get back on track with his exams do not appear to have been supported by staff at his school, indeed, it seems that even the Macmillan nurse's intervention was ineffective, thus suggesting some more effective liaison is needed to ensure that professionals outside the care setting continue the social support received within it.

However, it is not only the young adults with cancer who are affected by such disruption to their educational trajectory. Ross and his partner Hannah were living together when Ross was diagnosed with osteosarcoma. At the time he was self-employed, however, he appeared to be relatively sure that he would get his career back on track once he had completed his treatment and made a recovery:

I worked mainly for one company [that] was my . . . main customer. And I'll go back probably to just work for them full-time, I'd imagine, because they've been very understanding about my ability at the beginning, you know, what I mean, because I'm going to . . . tire easily and [be] weak and stuff, so they'll be understanding about it all.

(Ross)

The biggest disruption to plans appear to have affected Ross's partner Hannah who had withdrawn from university for a year in order to be with him throughout his treatment and to earn money to compensate for Ross's loss of earnings. She intended to return the following academic year but would be facing many of the same issues of seeing her friends having moved on a year or having graduated while she had suspended her studies. She had undertaken her support of Ross gladly, her commitment to him taking precedence over her degree. Nevertheless, this example shows that the impact on partners in this age group can be experienced in similar ways, the disruption of their own plans and life trajectory also being adversely affected.

At a slightly older age and with a more stable life style as the mother of a young child, Kelly, at 26, also experienced frustration, albeit slightly different from those expressed above:

> I used to like going up town, you know, and doing a bit of shopping, but I just couldn't do it. I just didn't have the energy to do it and I was stuck indoors and sometimes I thought she [her daughter] was going mad because she was stuck indoors. So it does have a big effect, you know, especially when you do have children as well, I think. I mean, my family is very good, you know. But at the end of the day, I mean, my mum's got bad arthritis, I can't expect her to run around after a 2-year-old, you know, because she's just full of energy is that one. We planned to go on holiday abroad and things like that, you know, and we had to cancel that and, you know, we used to like going for weekends away. Well, of course if I have treatment, you know, I don't feel like going away.
>
> (Kelly)

Kelly's daily activities such as going into town and visiting the shops were disrupted, so too were her family's plans for a holiday. Being incarcerated with a small child was also experienced as challenging, but Kelly did add that her daughter had forced her to focus on something other than her illness and had provided an imperative to get up every day and into activity. She was unable to give in to self-pity as she needed both to care about and to look after her dependent daughter. It could also be argued that while disappointed at not being able to go on holiday, such a loss did not represent the same disruption of Kelly's life trajectory as if she had been unable to take crucial exams, attend her first job interview or had been prevented from undertaking some of the more typical life stage activities that those in the younger age range had experienced as so frustrating. Thus here we can see how the effect of being slightly older with different responsibilities contrasts with the experiences of the young people who have not yet attained this infrastructure of stability, independence and identity.

While many of the accounts so far have been about the frustration of being prevented from living a 'normal' life, there can be a longer-term effect even after 'normal life' has been resumed. Steven, having felt deprived of the ability to enjoy himself during his illness and treatment, now lives for the day and as a result spends without much thought for the future:

Now if I want it, I just go out and get it, and that's the end of it ...
alright, I can't go out and buy anything and everything that I want,
but if I can afford it, then I just go out and buy it, and that's the end
of it, I don't worry about it. We don't pour thousands of pounds a
year into savings. Now, alright, that's probably a bit stupid but at the
minute it doesn't seem that important. I want to enjoy myself a little
bit now. I grew up quick, I grew from being an average 18-year-old
who wants to go out every Friday night, and every Saturday night
and get absolutely hammered and have a right good time, to, well, I
really can't do that now, I've got to take it a bit easy. I kind of feel a
bit deprived in some ways ... [there's] a gap I jumped a bit and that
was kind of annoying. Now I think I'm trying to go back the other
way. I should be thinking probably 'No, I should probably stay in and
save that money and put it in savings' now, it's like 'Ah, sod it, I've
got the money, I'm off out, I'm going to go out, I'm going to enjoy
myself.' Now whether that's right or wrong, I don't know, but it's
something I think I have to do. I have to try and get that little bit
back that I didn't have. 'Cause I couldn't really do anything for that
[time], sure, it was only a matter of a year or so, but I don't know, it
seemed to be a big bit, did that. There was a lot that I needed to do
that I didn't do. Or that I wanted to do that I didn't do and being
faced with the chance that you might not be able to do this, that's
the annoying bit.

(Steven)

It is clear from Steven's quote that he is attempting to regain some of what he
feels he missed out on and he is trying to cram as many experiences as he can
into his life to compensate. The year he was ill appeared to him to be a
considerable and significant percentage of his life and the frustration has left
him resentful at missed opportunities, but unlike Gemma who, in the last
chapter, we saw was saving carefully for an unpredictable future, Steven appears to be approaching money in a relatively cavalier fashion that is reminiscent of the way in which Mark 'blew' his windfall from the insurance
company (Chapter 4).

The impact on friendships

Many of the extracts thus far are about the disruption of plans and the dis-
appointment of not fulfilling aims and ambitions held perhaps throughout
childhood. However, to exacerbate the frustration, this is experienced at a
time of life when change is expected and indeed sought, and friends of the
same age are moving on to the next stage, leaving the young adult with

cancer feeling even more isolated and that life is passing them by while their friends are fulfilling their ambitions. This can be seen in the extract from Ruth's account:

> At times it seems as if the treatment regime for cancer is actually far worse than the disease itself and there have been times – especially in the dead of night – when I have wondered if my body could survive the effects of it all. (All this at a time, too, when all my friends were busy starting work on their GCSE courses and happily planning their futures!)
>
> (Ruth)

In Ruth's account we are reminded of Toni's comment that all her friends had gone to university while she was still going through treatment. The worry of the illness and the physical effects of both the illness and the treatment regimes are, as we can see from Ruth's comments, exacerbated by the knowledge that her friends were 'happily planning their futures'.

Getting back to normal and being with friends may be a relatively modest aim, yet, as Steven's experience shows, slotting back into the normal friendship groups may be difficult:

> Within a matter of weeks, really, you sort of really knew who your friends were. I lost a couple of friends – obviously I told them all, and a few of them were great, fine with it. You know, it's like, 'Well, you know, if ever, if you need owt, you just have to ask and that, and the job's a good un.' And everybody was alright initially but it was when the treatment started and I started feeling ill, generally. I remember one time I was home and a friend of mine turned up, well, I was ill . . . I wasn't well at all. And that was the last time I saw him . . . Yes, he never came back to my house or anything. I see him now at friends' parties and things like that, but we don't sort of talk really . . . I don't know whether he was scared . . . I don't really know. We never talked about it which sometimes I sort of regret really.
>
> (Steven)

Steven had been unable to understand the loss of his friend, yet his experience may not be unusual as it is closely mirrored by Mark's account that sheds some light on the difficulties encountered:

> I had a very close friend at the time that couldn't speak to me. He didn't know what to say . . . I talk to him now quite regular. And he just said he was totally lost for words, he was ten years older than me

... we were very, very close, more like brothers. And he said he just didn't know what to say, didn't know how to say anything to me.

(Mark)

It is interesting that Mark has been able to re-establish his 'lost' friendship and address the issue with his friend, but at 21, and with his friend being 10 years his senior this may have been easier than for those at the lower end of the age band. This is illuminated in the following quote from Ruth – much younger than Mark – in which we can see that even when the acute phase of the illness was over and 'normality' had been resumed, the illness had changed her in a fundamental way that separated her from her peers:

> When I went back to school, my friends were very glad to see me again but it was as if a curtain came down between us when I began to try to share the reality of the illness with them. It seemed that others had been advised not to 'hassle' me with questions about what I had been through – all very well meaning but not really what I wanted inside. I wanted to be able to speak about life as a cancer patient and life on the ward and what it feels like to be faced with a life-threatening illness. I know that I have been changed by what I have been through and that I am a different person now compared to a year ago and yet it seems that everyone expects me to go back to 'normal' as I was then. As my Macmillan nurse put it, it was as if I had had to grow up very rapidly and face real life and death issues while my peers were still coping with the normal teenage issues such as school work, relationships and increasing freedom. My priorities have changed radically as a result of having anaplastic large cell lymphoma and every day is now very precious to me – but along the way, it feels as if the illness has also opened up a rift between myself and many of my peers.

(Ruth)

There is a paradox here that while Ruth's plans for her future had been placed in doubt and on hold, at another level she had been catapulted into a degree of maturity that her peers cannot conceive of. To some extent the illness had already isolated her from the normal activities of the age group, it had delayed her plans, but it had also set her apart from her peers in a more profound way. Gemma too said, 'I feel older now.' This separation from and loss of friends are echoed by Devika who appeared to have lost touch with those she had considered to be close:

> Some people treated me differently because of my illness and even though we were in the same class and were like the best of friends, we sort of lost touch and barely spoke any more and now we have gone

our separate ways. Which is sort of hard for me as we were so close before and our relationships have changed so much in so little time. Well, let's just say that's when you find out who your true friends are.

(Devika)

Ricky's failed return to school was coupled with a wider social exclusion that was described by his mother as follows: 'Since the age of 15, he hasn't been a teenager. Boys go out with footballs and with girls, don't they, and they have a good time. He doesn't go out, he doesn't do anything.' Ricky continued by saying that all but one of his friends had 'deserted' him because he believed that they were scared and did not know what to say to him, but Ricky said: 'You just want people to talk to you normally.' Ross said that he had not heard from some of his friends since he had told them of his illness. He could not account for their lack of contact but thought they were scared of what they might see if they visited. Nevertheless, there were others who had stayed in contact, had visited, telephoned regularly and had also visited him in hospital. This was clearly of considerable importance to him.

The need for friends to maintain contact and lend a degree of normality to life was clear in the following comment from Charlotte:

I suppose you just need your family and your friends to be there when you need them and just carrying on treating you as normally as they can do really. Because that's the worst bit because you feel, like, I don't know, like an outsider.

(Charlotte)

Feeling like an outsider can be exacerbated by isolation from a peer group especially during a lengthy stay in hospital, and in many of the interviews the participants said that they just wanted to be treated 'normally', they did not want sympathy or pity, simply for life to be as 'normal' as it could be under the circumstances. The maintenance of friendships and reintegration into social life and education is a fundamental part of that normality, yet in Chapter 3 we saw accounts of resistance to allowing friends to visit during hospital treatment. This was recognized by the staff as unhelpful to sustaining friendships so necessary to reintegration during recovery, but we also re-member that in the last chapter Steven said that there were times that he did not want to be with friends and shut himself away in his bedroom.

However, the reluctance to encourage visits from friends may not only be felt by the young adult with cancer, their peer group may also feel uncertain about visiting. They are unlikely to be used to a hospital environment, and as a result may not have the confidence to arrange the visit themselves or if the hospital is at a distance they may have problems with transport. These life stage factors add to the likelihood of losing touch with friends, thus diminishing the peer support network and ease of adjustment back into 'normality' at a later stage. Thomas had needed to reassure his friends that they could still visit:

> Yeah, I miss my friends at the moment quite a lot because I've got quite a few friends back at school who come and visit me every now and then but I think they're OK, because the more they see me, the more they get sort of reassured, but I've been trying to tell them that I'm not always poorly, afterward [the chemotherapy] I'm alright and everything. I can still talk to them if they want to come and see me, so I think they've got a pretty good understanding of it now, but at the beginning they didn't know whether to come and see me or just stay away because they didn't know if I'd be well enough to talk to them.
>
> (Thomas)

In contrast, Hoody's friends had made considerable efforts to visit him and he spoke of how important this had been to his morale, particularly during his stay in hospital. Despite his friends living more than 60 miles from the hospital, they had nevertheless found ways to come as a group to support him during his lengthy stays on the specialist ward. Hoody had kept a photographic record of his cancer journey that included graphic depictions of every stage of the surgical removal of his bone tumour and much of the flesh and muscle surrounding it. While showing me these photographs, he also showed me ones of his friends surrounding his hospital bed, this tangible evidence of still being of importance and central to his friends' concern was clearly of great significance to Hoody. Interestingly, rather than try to conceal the enormity of his surgery and the physical scars, Hoody had sent copies of the surgical photographs to his school (where his mother taught) so that his fellow pupils could understand better what he had endured.

James' friends too were supportive, but James had initially feared their response to his illness; and again we see the importance of being treated as 'normal':

> Some of my friends from school came down to see me. I was so worried about what they would think about me and my situation, and how they would react to me. I was so grateful about how they were with me because they tried to treat me as normal as possible and spoke to me about football and what was going on at school, not just about my illness.
>
> (James)

Philip had stayed on at the Outward Bound centre during his convalescence, and this kept him in touch with his friends. However, he had to endure listening to them come back and recount the day's events and activities – a prospect denied to him for the foreseeable future:

> Well, the usual thing when people find out, they start trying to treat you differently so I soon made sure I put a stop to that. I just said, it's really not a big deal to me, I just made a joke with people about it, once they realized it really wasn't affecting me, they lightened up and they'd start cracking jokes about it as well and we'd have a laugh. Like I say, at the start, some people are a bit funny ... a bit too over-protective and things like that, you know. They always ask me, 'Oh, are you alright, you haven't done too much have you?' No, just treat me as normal ... [But] all my friends are doing [outdoor activities] and they come back talking about it. It was after my operation that was the hardest bit because I couldn't actually do anything, I had nothing going on in my life, I was just sat at home all day, every day, doing nothing, so I didn't have anything in common so much to talk to them about ... I used to drive out to where they were windsurfing and sit on the beach and watch ... still involved a little bit but that was sort of the hardest thing really, you know, from doing something all day every day to being told you can't do anything at all. I found that harder than finding out I was ill in the first place.
>
> (Philip)

Philip's experience of his friends accepting his altered status contrasts with Ruth and Devika's accounts, but Philip makes clear the distress he felt at being an outsider in his own world, so near and yet so far from the activities he loved, becoming literally an observer from the shore.

In the next quote we see that Gemma's friends' ability to support and understand her needs offers an even greater contrast to Ruth and Devika's experiences. However, Gemma was at the older end of the age group when diagnosed, and while frustrated at the need to abandon her plans to travel, it does seem that her friends had a degree of maturity that resulted in their ongoing support and friendship:

> My friends Laura, Toni and Elinor visited me, I was so glad. Laura is someone I have known since the start of college ... she is good at getting me to talk about awkward situations without me feeling I am unloading on her. She also suggested keeping a diary of the experience as a way of helping me understand the situation. Elinor is again very supportive and has a great sense of humour. Toni is the more controlled of all of us and keeps her feelings very close to her own heart, but she is a very stable friend ... without them I can't imagine what I would be like, their friendships are extremely important to me

... our get togethers are always lived to the full as they are rare due to us now living in different places and having busy schedules. These times when they came to me the tables felt turned as I am usually the one to sit down and talk about their problems, now I was the focus.

(Gemma)

The importance of Gemma's friends is clear; we recall that her family had emigrated to New Zealand, thus Gemma's reliance on them may have been of even greater significance, but she also indicates that her friends have moved away and are busy with their own lives.

So far, many of the accounts of friendships have focused mainly on the period during illness when activities have of necessity been limited. However, even when social activity is resumed, there are still limits on how easy it is to participate in the everyday 'taken for granted' events such as a barbeque:

There's stuff that I can't do and, like barbeques and things, because I have to watch what I eat in case there's any bacteria and things on it. When we go to barbeques we either take our own stuff or have like the salad stuff. And that's a bit annoying because I like my steaks medium rare, [but] I've got to have it cooked well through and that's difficult especially when you're going round to your friends. Because, like, the other day when I went to my friend from college to her house, and she said 'Do you want some tea?' I said, 'Yes, go on then.' And then she got all these take-away leaflets out, I had to say I can't have take-aways.

(Toni)

Similarly Ross and his partner Hannah, like James, found their lives constrained by the illness and his vulnerability to infection:

We try and live life as normally as possible, but obviously it's not like it used to be. You know, the biggest sort of thing, I have been looking quite well through all of my treatment, but not being able to mix with your friends and go out and socialize due to getting infections and stuff, that's one of the things that I found, find quite sort of difficult, is that you know staying at home and sort of hiding away from everybody. ... they'll ring up and [say] 'Shall we come round and see you?' [I'll say] 'You'd better not because I'm, you know, at a vulnerable time at the moment with low blood counts.' Like, for one occasion, like, we were going to go out for a meal ... but one of the relatives had a bit of an infection or something, so we didn't go because I was frightened of picking something up. Anyway we've had a few occasions like that haven't we?

(Ross)

We try not to look forward to anything too much.

(Hannah)

Whatever the friends' reactions, in all the examples above the young person had felt able to tell their friends about the cancer, yet Emma had not managed this, at least in part because she did not want to be treated differently. However, the effect on her life had not been to maintain the 'normality' of her relationships with friends, rather it seems to have resulted in despondency and isolation:

I don't talk about it ... not many people even know I've got it. None of my friends know ... nobody knows, I haven't told anyone ... because some people treat you differently. I don't want them doing that. I just expect them to find out from other people ... if I see people in the street, I talk to them, like, say, 'Oh, how are you?' and things like that, I just can't find the words to say 'Oh, yes, guess what, I've got cancer.' It's like I'm bragging about it or something. I just either hope that they already know or they'll find out. They probably won't believe me actually. I've stopped going out really. I'm too tired all the time. I can't be bothered to do anything. I just think.

(Emma)

We can see from these accounts that life plans are disrupted in many ways, from the relatively minor like not being able to eat a take-away meal, to the more major disruption of not being able to go to university or travel across the world on a long planned trip. Simon, the learning mentor for the TCT ward, was well aware of the fear of missed opportunities that the young people across the age band experienced, particularly in terms of their educational plans and the danger of losing ground that could not be caught up:

That's one of the consistent things through the whole age group. The ones who are at school have got quite a marked kind of way of telling whether they're falling behind their peers because they might miss a couple of months off school, go back, not know what their class is doing, realize that all their peers have moved on in their course work or their subjects and can notice they're behind. People who are at college or in between college and university, quite often see all their friends go off to university and they're stuck at home and, you know, perhaps they're not quite as free to go off and do that part of life as all their friends are. I think they really can feel the effects of that as well. I think it's very important actually across the whole age group again for them to keep in contact with their peers. Although their peers might be going off and doing some new and exciting things or they might be moving on at school, at least they've still got that link so they can still feel a part of that, part of that group.

(Simon)

The importance of encouraging and maintaining friendships is clear and is articulated with insight by Simon who is dealing largely with teenaged patients. The specialist ward is set up to minimize the disruption to education and career plans and to maximize the chances of social reintegration by encouraging friends to stay in contact. These are issues that will be addressed in terms of the policy for the provision of care in the final chapter.

Ongoing anxiety

The frustration at the disruption of plans so clear in the extracts above may be thought temporary, based on the assumption that after recovery from the illness 'normality' will be resumed. However, some participants who were beyond the acute illness stage and had begun their period of recovery, rebuilding their lives and carrying out their delayed plans indicated that they had been left with an underlying anxiety about their long-term health and their future. Steven's concern over symptoms that may or may not be sinister is clear in the following extract:

I don't really know how long [they] keep an eye on me for. Whether it's five, ten years . . . there are times, like at the minute I have a lump here . . . he's [the doctor] seen it and he says that's nothing because it goes up and down . . . he says that's obviously nothing to worry about. He knows it's just probably a little infection I've had. He says don't worry about that, that's nothing. And I'll sit there sometimes and just have my hand on my neck and I don't know whether . . . I do it out of habit more than anything, just sort of feel for any sort of lumps or bumps or whatever. And you don't sort of do it deliberately. You don't think 'Oh, Monday, oh, I'll give me neck a checking.' You don't think like that you just sort of do it . . . I got into the routine every week initially. It used to be Mondays, for instance . . . obviously I have to have a shower every day, in my job you're filthy . . . and Monday shower always check your neck. And that was the way it was, you know, but now I don't sort of say, 'oh, like, Monday again, shower and check me neck out.' Sometimes I'll be sat there watching telly and my hand will just go on.

(Steven)

Gemma too had been told that she was in remission but acknowledged that this does not mean she does not worry about a relapse:

On October 7th I had an appointment to find out my test results and everything is clear so far, so I'm in remission and now feel able to actually plan some of what I want to do in the future, like applying to work in New Zealand for six months which I had been planning before. I do feel I am still adjusting and I know that I will worry about the cancer returning but I do feel positive and very thankful that I was able to get to this point and I am healthy [but] I do worry about it coming back. But I know you can't worry about that all the time, I mean, I used to after the treatment. I think it was every hour that I thought about it. Now I probably still think about it every single day. Oh, I panic, yes. They're very, very happy with me ... they're quite confident ... it's completely gone but you always do have a wee bit of a worry.

(Gemma)

Gemma also said that she was concerned every time she had a cold or sore throat that the symptoms could herald a recurrence. Thus, despite the good prognosis, we see Gemma's underlying concern manifested by the qualification of her categorical statement about it 'being completely gone' with an admission that she always has a 'wee bit of a worry'. Despite several protestations about the treatability of her cancer, Kelly was still concerned that she might have a relapse:

One of the things that I always keep meaning to ask the consultant and I never do is, when you have cancer at such a young age, are you more prone to getting cancer when you're older? I mean, I know that lymphoma can come back again, but it is still very treatable ... I know it sounds awful but if you're going to have cancer, this is the one to have, because it is very treatable. But are you more prone to it in the future? I mean, I don't know and I suppose if I asked the consultant, he wouldn't either really. They don't like to say specifically, do they?

(Kelly)

Mark said that while he had been really 'positive about everything' during his illness, he became extremely anxious before a check-up:

I must admit if I'm going to a cancer appointment tomorrow, the
night before I'm a nervous wreck. I clean ovens. You can always tell
when I'm nervous because I clean the oven. I take the racks out of the
oven and that's what I do. And my wife says 'Why don't you come to
bed?' 'Oh, I can't yet, I've just got to do this.' I'm very positive on the
outside. Very nervous on the inside, I suppose. I've had three scares
in six years. I've got more lumps and they are something called
calcium stones. I have about thirty lumps at the moment. But they
are nothing. They can turn cancerous but on only rare occasions.
And they're being monitored of course.

(Mark)

When Mark is concerned about new lumps he calls the specialist who sees
him within three or four days and his fears are usually allayed. Yet despite his
admitted anxiety, Mark continued by saying that he knew he was going to be
fine. While this might be the case at a rational level, more than five years after
his initial diagnosis and with no recurrences, it is clear that at an emotional
level he is still deeply affected. We also saw in the last chapter that he always
wanted either his wife (preferably) or his mother with him at check-ups because of the 'one in ten thousand chance of it reoccurring and, and being told
on that day, and being on my own'.

It is not surprising that given the unthinkable had already occurred with
the development of cancer at this age, the prospect of its equally unthinkable
return continued to be a concern. Reassurances from health professionals
seem to have had only limited effect and though it was a minority of participants who raised their ongoing anxiety as an issue, this was likely to be due
to the fact that most were still in treatment at the time of the interview and
the prospect of life post-recovery appeared distant.

Discussion

Of course, illness at any age is likely to result in the disruption of plans and
life having to be put on hold while treatment and recovery take place, but
young adulthood is, as we have seen, characterized by impatience and a need
to move on to the next stage, to leave school, get a job, get qualifications, take
exams, go to university, or even just to have the kind of social life that is so
central to being young. Some of the examples of frustration presented here
may appear relatively mundane – after all, how important is a missed barbeque when compared to a life-threatening illness? Yet the distress at the loss
of the ordinary everyday activities was clear in the interviews. When control
has been lost in such a fundamental way, the additional small losses appear
much greater and are deeply symbolic. At the same time as their expectations

and plans – so long held – are put in jeopardy, the young person with cancer has to witness their peer group move on and away.

The issues raised in this chapter have direct relevance for policy and the provision of care. It is important that the ongoing educational needs of the young adults are addressed (Arbuckle et al. 2005), thus limiting the danger of falling behind with coursework. In the specialist care setting, personalized tuition can be made available, regardless of academic level (Geehan 2003). It is provided through the support of a learning mentor who has the resources not only to allow the young adults to keep up with academic work but who can also facilitate applications to university or assist with career choices. Such support is clearly of vital importance both during the illness and after recovery when the young adult is reintegrating and rebuilding their life.

It is clear that in the specialist care setting there is an awareness of the danger of losing touch with friends who are as a result encouraged to maintain contact (Morgan and Hubber 2004). According to Woodgate (2006), if included during the illness, special friends can be a source of enormous comfort to adolescents and both support and distract them through very difficult times, but social isolation 'may be driven by the sick teenager' (West Midlands Paediatric Macmillan Team 2005) so active measures may need to be taken to retain social contact. If this can be achieved, it will maximize the chance of reintegration that is a crucial part of the recovery process as social as well as physical recovery is central to the psychosocial well-being of the young adults. As Lewis (2005) says, maximizing the chances of survival should be accompanied by efforts to minimize the psychological and social cost of that survival and we have seen evidence in this chapter that the expertise in the specialist environment can indeed minimize the psychosocial damage. Thus, if professionals recognize the issues discussed in this chapter and can provide resources to meet the needs identified, this may help to alleviate some of the distress and disruption to the lives of the young adults thereby maximizing the possibility of compliance and recovery.

There is also evidence from the young people's accounts that future plans can be affected by an ongoing anxiety that is related to a fear of relapse and, as a result, continued support may be needed for some time after treatment and recovery (Neville 2000). However, this age group may not be well served by the standard services on offer (Zebrack 2006) so it may be that the only continuing support is offered by the specialist ward that goes on welcoming their discharged patients long after their treatment is over.

Key points

The interruption of the life trajectory results in:

- disrupted education – delayed university entrance and missed exams;

- missed job interviews and disruption to career plans;

- cancelled travelling;

- social isolation;

- loss of 'normality'.

Peer relationships suffer because friends:

- move on;

- move away;

- cannot cope;

- do not understand the constraints.

Ongoing anxiety is felt:

- with any slight ailment;

- before check-ups;

- over what the future holds;

- due to fear of infection;

- due to fear of relapse.

The specialist care setting can:

- facilitate educational and career plans;

- support contact with friends and encourage friends to visit;

- act as a vital life line to 'normality'.

6 The effect of the illness on physical appearance

As has been so powerfully demonstrated in the accounts from the young people in the previous chapter, the loss of normality, the disruption of their plans and their friends' continuing life trajectories combine with the physical symptoms and fears around the cancer and its effects to make a uniquely challenging set of circumstances. When these factors are combined with changing physical appearance, morale can be lowered even further.

The effect of the illness on their appearance was raised as an issue by almost all of the participants in the research. This is unsurprising, as Lewis (2005: 242) acknowledges, 'self-image is pivotal to normal development' and this is endorsed by Hain (2005) who says that adolescents are immensely sensitive to their physical appearance and that this is a time when even minor blemishes can be considered disastrous to a healthy adolescent (West Midlands Paediatric Macmillan Team 2005). Larouche and Chin-Peuckert (2006) argue that the body changes that take place during adolescence lead to a preoccupation with looks that is coupled with a tendency for adolescents to compare themselves to how others look. According to Craig:

> A physical appearance that the young person feels identifies them as different from everyone else may cause feelings of being damaged and deviant in the outside world, further contributing to feelings of low self esteem. At a time when peer group acceptance and support is so important, they may feel increasingly ostracized.
>
> (2006: 113)

As Brannen et al. (1994) say, 24 per cent of all young people are dissatisfied with their body image and nearly half of all young women have tried to lose weight. So we can see that appearance is central to youth culture and any threat to it can jeopardize confidence and a sense of belonging and identity. The illness and treatments associated with cancer frequently result in adverse changes to body image and can manifest in hair loss, weight loss, weight gain and scars from surgery which, as a result, leave young adults ill at ease in social situations (Arbuckle et al. 2005). Zebrack charts graphically the possible adverse effects on physical appearance:

Alterations in physical appearance, including weight changes, hair loss, amputations, placement of catheters ... scars and alterations in skin coloration and texture, not only make children and teens feel different from peers but may also represent frightening changes in the body with an adverse impact on self esteem. Fears that the body will never return to its original appearance, of not being recognized by others or of being mistaken for an individual of the opposite sex, often lead to shame, social isolation, and regressive behaviours ... chemotherapy and radiation treatments sometimes make patients feel as if their bodies are not their own.

(2006: 224)

Zebrack continues by saying that for adolescents the adverse effects on their appearance are more of a problem than the pain of treatments. The impact of such physical change is powerfully demonstrated in this extract from Ruth's account:

My hair had by now almost completely fallen out and was every-where – on the pillows, the sheets, the floor. ... I dread to think what my friends at school would say if they could see me now – even I found it hard to believe that this was really me! (I wonder – could it be a deliberate oversight that there is no mirror in Cubicle C!)

(Ruth)

In this short paragraph Ruth captures a number of challenges that in addition to the illness itself can make life so problematic for young adults with cancer. This is a time of life when appearances assume enormous importance, many magazines for young people, particularly girls, focus on clothes, hair, make-up and body shape. Fashion can be used as a statement that situates young people in a peer group and image is a way of beginning to establish an identity at a formative life stage. Peer relations are integral to adolescent identity and as Neville (2000: 9) says, this identity is closely related to 'sameness' and this is manifested by a preoccupation with dress, appearance and body image which are intrinsic to identity.

It is therefore unsurprising that many of the young people in the research expressed considerable distress about the changes in their appearance; indeed, for some it seemed to have a greater impact than the illness itself. In Chapter 3 we have already seen that some of the young people did not want their friends to visit them in hospital at least in part because of the way they looked.

There was a tendency for the young women to focus on appearance more than the young men, but there is evidence in the following accounts that young men are also badly affected by the impact on their appearance.

Nevertheless, this chapter begins with a quote from a young woman. Gemma was 23 at the time she was diagnosed with Hodgkin's lymphoma; the lengthy passage from her narrative account has been selected and presented in its entirety as it addresses many of the issues with power and clarity:

> I had organized a hair appointment to cut off my long hair in preparation. I felt awful, but pushed myself to get up and meet my friend Toni who was my moral support. I have never had short hair and I loved my hair. My hairdresser is great and remembers you with each visit. I explained why I needed it cut, it's recommended so the shock of it falling out isn't so much. She understood totally as she had done the same for her mother when she had to go through chemotherapy. I cried when the first bit was cut, then gathered myself. My friend sat next to me throughout, I was so grateful for that support. My hairdresser told me about other clients who have gone through losing their hair and then it coming back thicker and curly. When she had finished, I hated it, it wasn't the cut, which was great, I didn't like the way I looked, but my friend told me it looked good. Eventually I came round to it. I went shopping for an outfit for my Christmas works do the next day with Toni. I got one but I nearly passed out in the changing rooms and so went home. I had pushed myself too far and felt rougher than I had ever felt in my life ... nausea and a feeling I just can't describe other than the worst hangover you could ever have.
>
> Boxing Day [in hospital] and my hair started to fall out; although I was prepared for this no one can prepare you for how you feel about it and how horribly it falls out. [As] I had cut my hair short in preparation [I] was hoping my hair [would] only thin. My hair was incredibly itchy and it was slowly driving me mad. I was watching TV and my hair was falling out all over the chair, the floor, just everywhere. The cleaner came in and it was swept up, I was shocked at seeing it all. I was getting increasingly upset and was trying to stay calm in front of the staff, but I felt like screaming and crying. I mentioned it to one of the staff and they said that I could shave it if it would feel better. Shave my hair! I realized now I was so underprepared for this...
>
> I found the physical changes through my treatment hard to take. Throughout my chemo I managed to put on a stone and a half. I had gone from a size 10 to only just being able to fit into size 12 clothes. I had hardly any clothes to wear and didn't feel like shopping for them either. I felt huge and bloated and had never been this heavy in my life. I suppose it was hard to deal with as no one had told me this could happen, I thought I would lose weight. Also due to the steroids

my face became round, which made me feel even worse as it showed off my weight. The fact I had no hair to cover this made it even more prominent. I had opted not to have a wig; I think I would have been more conscious of people noticing. I wore bandanas and ended up having 26 in the end, people were going on holiday and sending me different ones and if I saw a different one in a shop I would buy it. Going out in a bandana is an interesting experience, people tend to look at you more as you stand out. To start with, this was an uncomfortable experience and it made me not want to go out of the house but I eventually got used to [it] and didn't care as much. I never took them off, not even to sleep as I didn't want anyone else to see. I think at one point I went through a very bad patch and couldn't manage to look in the mirror when I would take it off for a shower. I felt I looked like a freak and said it frequently – 'bald-headed freak'. It's not the best attitude to have but I was mourning my old image, my hair. The hair on my legs and underarms slowed, this was an upside to the treatment. Oh, and the free Brazilian, no one tells you about that!

There had been lots of new pubs opening and so [I] wanted to go round a few that were new ... I was stopped at the door and asked to remove my bandana. I laughed as I thought this was a joke and carried on walking, he then stopped me and said to take off my bandana, as there was a 'no headgear' policy. I turned round and explained that I was wearing it due to having chemo and had lost my hair and that I don't want to remove it. He was insistent that we couldn't go in, I was so angry that I just walked away feeling totally humiliated. I could have understood if I'd had hair underneath it or if it had something offensive written on it but it was black with white flowers on it. My friends stayed behind and argued with him, I called back to them to just leave it. My confidence about my appearance was low enough, I didn't need someone being that insensitive and stupid.

I get angry that I am never going to be who I was before all of this happened, I will never have that life again and it is going to take so long to look how I want to look again. I know physicality isn't the most important part of life but it is an important part of how I present myself and how I am comfortable. I don't feel confident in the way I look anymore and I know this is something I will have to get used to in the short term. The weight is coming off and the hair is growing, just not fast enough. Back to the clothes – I basically was not prepared with how much my new hair changed the way I would buy clothes. I can't wear skirts or dresses as I look, to me, not feminine enough. I got upset with myself when I tried one on and felt like going home straight away. I was in the middle of Debenhams and couldn't cry, but if I could have, I would have done. Thank goodness for Toni who was with me, she just linked arms with me and continued looking with me with patience I had never recognized before. I ended up buying something that I would have never worn before as it didn't suit my previous shape. Although I didn't get the same excitement out of the shopping, as I would have done previously, it did show me once again how much support I still need.

(Gemma)

This account raises many issues that demonstrate the impact on self-confidence and emotional well-being. Clearly concern over physical appearance is at the heart of many of Gemma's observations, and these have had a profound effect on her sense of identity so that even when Gemma's body shape began to return to 'normal', she felt that the other and more lasting changes still fundamentally challenged her identity, who she was – or who she appeared to be – to the extent that even when her original clothes fitted her again, they no longer looked 'right'.

In addition to the sense of grief for the person she felt she had lost through the illness and treatment, is the knowledge that she is judged by others on the physical appearance she presents and that this can result in public humiliation. However, what is also clear in this extract is the importance of her friend Toni. The effect on friendships was addressed in the last chapter. In Gemma's case we can see that rather than feeling her friends were moving on without her or marginalizing her from social activity, they continued to support her. This may be because, at 23, she was older than some of the participants and her friends were more mature. The quote also demonstrates the centrality of friends' contribution to emotional recovery from the effects of the illness, and thus the importance of maintaining contact throughout the potentially isolating period during hospitalization and treatment. Yet we also remember that in Chapter 3 these same friends had been reluctant to visit Gemma in hospital lest they should bring germs.

Charlotte who had also lost her hair and put on weight articulated the necessity of friends' support to provide her with the confidence to go out, but in her case it seems that not all her friends understood this need. The result for Charlotte was that she tended only to go out with her mother and with one good friend who she saw on a weekly basis:

I think you need your friends and they just look at you different because, like, you've lost your hair or whatever. They think, 'Oh, well, I won't speak to her or I'll just ignore her' ... Well, I don't go out as much because I won't go out on my own ... if I have to walk to the shop, I don't like going on my own because people look at me and that. Whereas if I'm with someone else, I can ignore them looking at me so I like to go with someone else.

(Charlotte)

However, it was not only the young women who were concerned about weight gain. James at 16 found his treatment upsetting not only because it made him 'very-short tempered and angry' after which he felt guilty that he had 'moaned at everyone', it also made him put on a lot of weight which distressed him.

Nicola said that her appearance, particularly at first, had prevented her feeling that she could go out and socialize with her friends primarily because of her hair loss. She eventually overcame that inhibition but told the following story about a trip out with friends:

> I ended up thinking, 'Well, sod it, if anybody's going to say anything then I will put them straight'. I . . . went into Bolton town centre for a party and a friend of mine got rather tiddled, and she was holding on to me. And as we were walking back to the car, this bloke turned round and said, 'Oh, you dyke', and I turned round and said, 'Well, if you think I'm a dyke, then heaven help you.' And he sort of looked at me very odd and I said, 'I can't wait until you start losing your hair at forty.' And I walked away because . . . I just thought no, it's not fair to be so rude just because a friend of mine is drunk and she's holding on to me and I have no hair. You have the right to call me something like that? That's very stereotypical.

(Nicola)

This account is reminiscent of Gemma's in that strangers encountered on a night out with friends felt able to make comments based on an appearance that was perceived as in some way 'socially unacceptable'. It appears that in neither case was there awareness on the part of the casual observer that the hair loss was the result of illness and chemotherapy, but rather provoked an assumption that the young women were flouting social conventions, thus making them 'fair game'. It is perhaps more likely for others to criticize openly or attack verbally people in this age group than either children or older adults. This may be because the lack of hair, or even scars, are interpreted as a fashion or life style statement relating to youth culture and thus perceived as threatening and this 'legitimates' the resulting hostility. As Alison (the lead cancer nurse outside the specialist setting) recognized:

> It's the stigma . . . I've had people come to me and say . . . that they were in bank queues and could hear other people, 'Oh, why [has] that person had their head shaved like that? Don't they look ridi-

culous?' and 'Look at that person there with the scars on their arms' where they've had multiple phlebotomies ... I think if you see an adult with a very short haircut, many people now will think 'I wonder if that's person's undergone chemotherapy?' Whereas, if you see an adolescent they think it's a fashion statement.

(Alison)

Nicola recollected the first time she felt confident enough to take off her bandana in public:

> I remember I went down to Milton Keynes to see a friend from boarding school. And I'd gone down on the train and had my bandana on, and was quite self-conscious sat in the train sort of reading my book and hiding away in a corner. And I got off the train, she [my friend] gave me a big, big hug and said, 'Oh, you're looking lovely', and that made me feel quite good. Then she said, 'We're going out tonight, do you want to come out with us?' I said, 'Oh, yes, of course, I would, it would be lovely', and she said, 'Why don't you take your bandana off'? I went, 'No, no, no, no, no. I don't, don't want to take my bandana off', but she said, 'You've got hair, it is only baby soft, but you've got hair.' And it was the very first time I took my bandana off and actually went out without it on, which was great. It made me feel so good, and all these random guys are going round touching my head and going 'Oh, you're like a little baby.' It was great and it made me feel a lot better, and they didn't ask any questions until obviously later on. They were getting to know me and they were like 'So how, how come?' And I'd sit and say, 'Well, it's because of cancer that I've lost my hair.'

(Nicola)

Nicola's account is resonant of what Larouche and Chin-Peuckert (2006: 206) call a 'peer-shield'; that is the strong, caring attitude of friends that, rather than isolating the young adult with cancer, acts a protective shield from criticism and negative comments.

Emma's distress in anticipation of losing her hair had been one of the factors that had contributed to her refusal to be treated for several months. She felt that she had been offered little support in the non-specialist setting and that her partner Gary did not understand her distress because as she put it: 'It's alright for him because he's a man.' It was only when she was referred to a specialist ward that the support she was offered made the prospect acceptable:

I wanted to not have any treatment. I wanted to delay it for ages so I'd have my hair for longer . . . I wanted to go on holiday and things like that but I can't do things like that because I don't know how long I'm going to have my hair. I don't want to go on holiday with no hair. [At the non-specialist ward] they don't really talk to you about nothing. Oh, they said, I could go get a wig which was quite good. I went to do that. But you had to choose between two . . . there was loads and loads and loads on the table I wanted to try some more on. I think she was pushed for time because she was late, because she had people waiting outside as well.

(Emma)

Many of the young women assumed that the loss of their hair was not as bad for the young men. Emma and Adrian's partner's mother both suggested that young men might be less affected by the loss of hair as they tend to wear caps. Some of the other female participants said the same as did members of staff; for example, Deborah a staff nurse on the TCT ward, said of young men: 'Obviously there's less likelihood that the hair loss is going to bother them. They just wear caps or whatever.' While mourning her own changing appearance and hair loss, it is clear that Nicola assumes that a young man would not find it as distressing:

You start losing your hair, which is a horrible thing, especially as a woman, it's not as bad for young blokes. Especially when it's the football season because they've all shaved their heads anyway, so it's not a big deal. But young girls, no hair doesn't look right, it doesn't seem right at all. But daft things like going to the shop, I'd have to get myself ready. There's putting your make-up on . . . drawing your eyebrows on, drawing your eyelashes on, putting your cap on or your bandana, and putting on rosy cheeks so you make yourself look as healthy as possible. Even though you look like a hamster because of the amount of drugs and everything you've had pumped into your system and steroids . . . you ended up sort of with teeth at the top of your cheeks.

(Nicola)

Although young women may be confronted with particular challenges in terms of their appearance, their assumption about the equanimity with which hair loss is accepted by the young men is not supported by my interview data. This is shown in the following quote from Adrian. Talking of his hair loss he said:

> When I was out with my friends they'd always say, 'Take your hat off we're not bothered, we're not bothered' ... they used to hide my hat around the pub and say 'You know, you're our friend, we're not bothered what you look like.' They said, 'It's what's inside, you're our friend. We know you're not well so why are you hiding it sort of thing ...' But then ever since then I've started wearing a hat every day. As soon as I get out of bed it's straight on ... if you're walking through town you could see people staring at you, having a good look and ... yes and because of my age really I think ... they don't expect to see it [baldness] and when they do see it it's like 'Oh my God.' So really I just wore a hat and then that was it, I've just worn a hat since ... now I wear it constantly, I never go out without my hat.
>
> (Adrian)

It is interesting that despite Adrian's friends specifically telling him that they were not bothered about his appearance and it was 'who he was' rather than 'what he looked like' that mattered to them, he still felt a compulsion to wear a hat. At the time of his interview, Adrian's hair had grown back fully – though he told me it was different in colour and texture, but he still insisted on wearing a hat at all times, including during the interview. Adrian was interviewed in his home which he shared with his partner Cindy's parents. When Cindy's mother joined the discussion, she said that she had got quite used to him with no hair and that to her he had looked stranger when it had started to grow back She also said that 'Young lads wear caps and that now ... it's not like a woman losing all her hair.' The fact that Adrian had kept his eyebrows was thought to be beneficial, as Cindy's mother said of losing eyebrows: 'sometimes that makes you look really strange, doesn't it?' While I was talking with Cindy's mother, Adrian went to fetch a photograph of him and Cindy taken during his treatment. I commented on what a lovely photograph it was, Cindy's mother agreed but Adrian said he didn't like any of the photos that had been taken of him while he was ill.

Nathan too was deeply distressed by his hair loss:

> If I had my hair, I'd have a lot of confidence. And if I had my colour back and stuff like that, I'd have a lot more confidence ... you can talk to people better. You're not as shy. But with this, losing my hair and stuff like that it, it has knocked my confidence. Because people say I used to have, like, a big head, I'm big-headed and stuff, but now it's like [I'm] small-headed. I don't think much of myself and it isn't fair. That's all I can say.
>
> (Nathan)

It is clear from Nathan's account that the loss of his hair had a profound effect on his sense of confidence, and we remember from Chapter 3 that he refused to allow even close friends to visit because of his appearance. It seems that his earlier reputation for being 'big-headed' in a sense of being a big personality, had transformed quite literally into being, as he puts it, 'small-headed'. He had lost both his hair and confidence together, making his head and personality feel small to him, though probably to no one else. Similarly Hoody reflected on the effect that his changing appearance had when he went out:

> The last time I went into town, I had a tube stuck up my nose, I didn't have any hair, I looked awful, I was pale, like. And sometimes people just stare at you and everyone just looks at you. And when, when you're in a wheelchair you're getting pushed around and people don't realize you're there and you know you've got to, like, say 'Excuse me, excuse me' all the time.
>
> (Hoody)

Coupled with Hoody's discomfort about his appearance was the added ignominy of being pushed in a wheelchair. For a previously strong athletic young man, this seems to have been experienced as humiliating. Paradoxically, in addition, he felt both conspicuous in that people stared at him while also being rendered 'invisible' by being ignored and being 'pushed around', both literally and metaphorically.

So it seems that assumptions made by the young women about the relatively advantageous position of young men in relationship to hair loss were unfounded. Far from feeling advantaged by the social acceptability of being able to wear a cap, some of the young men interviewed said that the fact that women could wear wigs was an advantage of being female, but that it would be totally unacceptable for them as men to consider a wearing a wig. Yet this male assumption about the young women was in most cases as misguided as the young women's assumptions about the men. For example, Dawn never felt comfortable or confident in her wig:

> I was convinced it looked like a wig ... when I put my wig on ... I don't know if it was because I knew it was a wig, and I got it into my head that it was a wig. I didn't have the confidence to wear it. But I just wore bandanas ... because they were in at that time.
>
> (Dawn)

Toni also said that for her 'The worst thing was the losing the hair' though she had enjoyed choosing a wig:

> They said: 'Oh, but you'll definitely lose your hair.' And ... it just hit me and I just burst into tears and it was quite hard. Because it didn't

happen until this second treatment and then it started coming out quite a lot and that was quite difficult. But when I went for my wig, it was really fun ... But my friends and friends' mums, like, they always thought that if anything like this happened, I'd shave it off because I wouldn't be able to deal with it. That's just the one thing I couldn't do. It's, like, if you think of shaving your hair off and you go ... [shudder] I'd [rather] let it thin out and gradually get used to it.

(Toni)

Although, unlike Dawn and Gemma, Toni had opted for a wig, had selected one that she really liked which resembled her own hair and was reminiscent of a favourite style, she nevertheless had insecurities about it:

The only thing about it is when you're walking round you have to be careful because it might slip back a bit or ... I have to get my mum to sort it out sometimes because sometimes when I do it, it just looks like you're wearing a wig. So I get my mum to sort it out and then it looks alright ... I'm paranoid of like walking down a street and it flying off or something like that. Because when she [mother] was brushing once, she went like that [gesticulates] and it just flew off my head.

(Toni)

Even when hair begins to grow back, as Devika pointed out, it may not be the same as before the chemotherapy – as with Adrian's – additionally, there may be other lasting physical changes that can continue to affect levels of confidence:

There are also a few things that have gone wrong in my life since then, like relationships, my hair and my height ... the treatment, which I got made me lose my hair, which, as a girl, is a very big deal. Although it is sort of growing back, it isn't really growing properly and is sort of thin in places. This is horrible for me and is extremely annoying. Another thing, as I said before, is my height. I have sort of stopped growing and I'm kind of small for my age, which I also hate.

(Devika)

Kelly, the oldest of the participants at 26 was not so concerned about her hair; rather, it was the weight gain that she had found more difficult to tolerate:

I put a lot of weight on with the steroids ... I mean, I've put on so much weight and ... was talking to the consultant last week ... and I said, 'You know, I'm not happy about all this weight I'm putting on.'

I mean, I can't stop eating. You know because it triggers your appetite and I just could not stop eating. And I used to sit there thinking 'You don't need it.' But I couldn't help it. So I've put all this weight on. And I said to him, 'I'm not happy.' So he took me off the steroids and I felt so much better ... I'm not bothered about the hair. I mean thankfully I've got a lot of hair but it has thinned out, but even if it all went, I wouldn't have bothered so much ... I went to a wedding in October ... I had my outfit but because I'd had it for ages I had to squeeze into it and I felt so uncomfortable and so self-conscious because I'd put all this weight on. And I just didn't enjoy the day because I just thought, 'Oh God, you know, I'm sure I'm hanging out all over.' ... That's what was really bothering me the most because I kept saying, 'Oh, look how much weight' and everyone's going, 'Yes, but you can't help it.' I say, 'Yes, I know, but it's horrible you know.' 'Oh, you'll lose it all when you're all done.' ... it's all right saying that but you don't feel that at the time, do you know what I mean, you think, 'Oh God.' So I have to breathe in a bit more.

(Kelly)

We can see that Kelly is just as concerned and depressed about her weight gain as any of the younger participants. Her friends appear to have been supportive and reassuring, though their comments do not seem to have made her feel any better about her appearance and her self-consciousness at the wedding is clear. The effect the weight gain has had on her relationship with her husband will be discussed in the next chapter.

While Ross had also put on weight and lost his hair, this did not appear to be of much concern to him, indeed, he seemed to be quite confident despite the physical effects of the illness and treatment, nevertheless, he was taken aback not to be recognized by his work mates:

I looked at a picture of myself from like a year or two ago and I thought, 'Oh, I do look a bit different.' Like, you know, obviously hair loss and stuff ... being bald doesn't bother me ... You know, I've had two fingers and half of my arm amputated and it doesn't bother me showing people ... and if people want to have a look they can have, can have a look, I don't mind. But I went up to a place where I worked a couple of months ago just to see everybody and there was a guy there who I've worked with for about three years, like not every day but on and off and [I was] quite close friends with him. And he was a little distance from me just across the yard and I said 'Hello' and he sort of went 'Alright' ... He never recognized me at all. I was a bit surprised ... I wasn't really upset by it or anything but I was a bit surprised I thought, 'Surely I don't look that much different.' But I

> suppose with no hair and I've put weight on, I'd be a bit chubbier round the chops a bit more than I used to be.
>
> (Ross)

Not being recognized by others is one of the fears charted by Zebrack (2006), but this seems to have been dealt with relatively well by Ross who was also sanguine about the change in his appearance. However, he was in a long-term committed relationship that provided a degree of stability and security, and this might have contributed to the apparent equanimity with which he accepted the changes in his appearance. Nevertheless, Kelly was also in a secure relationship but far less accepting of such change, thus it may be that there is an element of gender difference in the ability to tolerate an altered appearance.

Most of the physical manifestations of the illness discussed thus far have been those that could be seen by the casual observer, yet there are also other 'hidden' changes that may not be apparent to anyone else but which clearly affect confidence. Mark told me of the insecurity he had felt about having his testicle surgically removed:

> I had false testes put in which give me a lot of confidence [but] I struggled with infection, it kept swelling up and going back down ... at first they thought it might have been the false testicle rejecting, like, not wanting to be in there ... but fortunately it settled down because there was talk of removing it at one stage. [If they had re-moved it] I would never have gone swimming in a pair of shorts and got out of the water with people ... there's always something in the back of your mind that somebody might look and say, 'Oh, he's hanging funny, him.' But 99.9 per cent probably would never even notice. But just for your own peace of mind.
>
> (Mark)

However, Mark acknowledged that his father who had also had testicular cancer and had a testicle removed without opting for a prosthetic replace-ment went swimming with him every two weeks, yet neither he nor his father ever considered this to be problematic. Again this suggests that the issue for a young man is perceived and experienced differently.

Simon, the learning mentor on the TCT ward, said the following about his observations of the impact on appearance and resulting effect on the willingness to allow friends to visit:

> From what I can tell, it's quite rare that friends actually come in, probably across the whole age group, but the younger ones, I think, their friends find it very difficult ... Because obviously the patient's

appearance changes quite a lot, and can change quite rapidly from losing a lot of weight, because of not being able to eat, then putting on lots of weight on things like steroids and things which really can increase your size. So I think it's quite hard for friends. And there's hair falling out, and things like that really change someone's appearance. I think friends can find that quite difficult . . . some of them have said explicitly to friends, 'Don't come and visit me, I don't want you to, don't want you to see me in here, and I'll see you when I'm at home and feeling better' . . . a lot of people seem to think that the girls find it more difficult than the boys with hair loss, but I've not really found that especially true from the patients that I've had contact with . . . they do all find it difficult on some level but I think the girls have quite a lot of support with hair loss and things. They have quite a lot of nice wigs and different hats and things. Whereas, the boys, it's kind of a skin head or a baseball cap and that's about all you've got and I don't know it can be quite obvious that there's a bald head underneath there with some of the hats that they wear, I think they can find that, they can find it quite tricky.

(Simon)

It is clear that Simon recognizes the profound impact of the change in appearance and understands that boys may find hair loss as traumatic as do the girls, but that the boys do not necessarily receive the support they need to manage the loss. He also makes an observation on the reluctance to allow friends to visit which is reminiscent of Nathan's comment in Chapter 3 that because of his appearance he did not want his friends to see him in hospital as he feared this would alter their future relationships after he had recovered. However, as we saw in the last chapter, and through some of the quotes in this chapter, if friendships can be maintained, they can be of great support throughout the illness and also can assist in reintegration into social life and the 'normal' activities of young adulthood during recovery.

Discussion

The data show that the change of appearance brought about by the illness and its treatments has a profound effect on the morale and self-confidence of the young people. In Emma's case, so great was her distress at her potential hair loss that she would have refused treatment had she not been referred to a specialist unit, thus demonstrating how crucial sensitive and effective communication by staff is at ensuring compliance and possibly survival. Yet, according to Shaw et al. (2004), healthcare professionals' ability to communicate effectively with young people with cancer, whose body image is fragile, is very limited. This may be the case particularly outside the specialist setting where the psychosocial aspects of the illness are not so well understood and difficulties in communication are exacerbated by a lack of expertise in knowing how to engage with the young adults in an area they find so distressing.

According to Hedstrom and von Essen (2004), while parents recognized that their children had experienced altered self-image as particularly distressing, only one nurse mentioned this as an issue in relationship to a single child. It is interesting to note that the children in Hedstrom and von Essen's study were younger than adolescents at between 4–7 years; nevertheless, even at their age, body image was of considerable significance. In a reflection from a social worker's perspective, Arbuckle et al. suggest that training is essential for staff who may lack confidence, and it should include awareness in the area, as young people may tend to minimize the physical effects out of 'embarrassment, invincibility or fear' (2005: 239).

There is a tendency to assume that hair loss in particular is a greater problem for the young women than for the young men. Indeed, the young men and women themselves each assumed the other gender had it 'easier' in some sense, yet, as we have seen, both young men and young women were affected in a very similar way. Despite the age range from Ruth at 14 to Kelly at 26, the issues were similar, again suggesting that there is more that unites those across the age range than that which divides them. While it is likely that a person of any age will be distressed at a negative impact on their appearance, it seems that for children or for much older adults, the effects will be mitigated by other factors. The amount of socializing done during teenage years and young adulthood coupled with the importance of appearing fashionable and part of a peer group all combine to make the experience of changing appearance more challenging to this age group. This may be exacerbated, as we have seen, by the stares and offensive comments made by casual passers-by – again a phenomenon that might be less likely with either children or older adults.

'Appearance' may be a personal issue and seem at first sight to be unrelated to policy or outcomes. However, professionals' recognition of the trauma endured when appearance is changed or damaged, coupled with practical support in offering strategies to minimize or address the physical changes and deal with the distress may result in the young cancer patient being more willing to undergo radical or aggressive treatment. One of the strategies can be to offer a workshop run by volunteer beauticians that help to enable the teenagers look their best and which give them 'tremendous self confidence' (Robertson 2006). Additionally, recognition of the social stigma and misunderstanding that may result from hair loss can be addressed through the provision of a card supplied by the specialist unit and carried by the young person to show at night clubs where entry may otherwise be denied. These practical interventions and the support offered for the management of the detrimental effects on appearance may increase the likelihood of compliance and, by extension, survival. In addition, the increased confidence from such support may also contribute to a willingness to let friends visit and to lessen concern about the impact their appearance will have outside the confines and relative safety of the care setting.

We also remember from Chapter 3 that being treated in a specialist facility alongside a peer group undergoing similar physical effects on their appearance created an environment where the young people were more at ease with showing their physical changes without a need to disguise them. As reintegration after treatment is central to social as well as emotional recovery, any chance of building confidence that can carry the young adult through to the next stage should be embedded into practice that runs alongside the medical treatments.

Key points

The impact on appearance is of fundamental significance because:

- body image is central;

- boys and girls are equally affected;

- appearance signifies belonging;

- identity may be threatened;

- self-confidence may be damaged;

- abuse/taunting may be experienced;

- rejection may be feared;

- social isolation may result;

- compliance may be affected.

---

7 Sexuality and fertility

The accounts in the last chapter have clearly shown the effect of illness and treatment on morale and self-esteem when appearance is altered. As we have seen, this can have a negative impact on confidence levels when socializing in general. This chapter continues that theme by examining the impact that the cancer experience has on sexual relationships, both those already established at the point of diagnosis and those yet to be formed. As Craig says:

> Much normal adolescent activity and discussion is focussed on sexual awareness, finding a partner, and sexual activity. Through peer group isolation, young people with life-limiting illness often miss out on this normal adolescent information and discussion.
>
> (2006: 112)

Here Craig is referring to young people with a wide range of illnesses that include those that are congenital, which may have limited the young person's opportunity to have had a sexual relationship. However, young adults with cancer will face many of the same issues, though, in their situation, relationships that pre-date the cancer may have been thrown into crisis by the illness, the change in their appearance and their physical isolation in hospital. As Nishimoto (1995) points out, having cancer does not eradicate sexual urges and the result may be distressing for the young person who may have to come to terms with the possibility of future intimate relationships being threatened. This may have far-reaching consequences. Sexuality is particularly closely related to self-regard; feeling able to evoke desire in another person results from positive feelings and beliefs about one's own personality and physical appearance (Grant and Roberts, 1998; Quinn 2003). Accordingly, the physical changes of the disease may make the adolescent feel that he/she is not sexually attractive (West Midlands Paediatric Macmillan Team 2005: 139).

Yet according to Shaw et al. (2004: 144–5), healthcare professionals often fail to make the link between issues of body image and sexuality, additionally, these authors claim that 'discussing sexual issues is a vital area often neglected or avoided by nurses' because they are embarrassed, lack the appropriate knowledge or assume that this issue should be left to doctors. According to Balen and Glaser (2006), adolescents may also have difficulties raising their concerns about both sexual function and reproduction with their doctors. As Kline (2006: 175) points out, up until the point of diagnosis, particularly at the younger end of the age range, the patient has focused on 'being a "child" and has not thought about the prospect of future fertility' which they subsequently find difficult to initiate as a topic of discussion. As a result, the anxieties experienced by the young adults may well remain un-addressed as no one raises the issue and attention focuses on the illness and its treatment which in any case tends to be the immediate concern for staff and parents.

The difficulties with sexual relationships can be exacerbated by the effects of the illness and its treatment which can jeopardize fertility in both the young men and the young women. At an age when they are unlikely to have yet had children, this can have a devastating effect. As Zebrack (2006) says, young adult survivors' sense of self and of normality is bound up at least in part with a belief in their ability to have children of their own; yet according to Reebals et al. (2006), between 15–30 per cent of cancer survivors are left permanently sterile following therapy. In addition, Wallace and Brougham (2005) say that gonadal damage and resulting infertility can be caused not only by chemotherapy and radiotherapy, but also by the disease itself. For example, they say that 70 per cent of male patients with Hodgkin's disease assessed before they begin treatment are found to have impaired semen quality. Wallace and Brougham argue, opportunities for preserving fertility must be grasped, and all male patients who are able to produce semen should have the chance to bank sperm before treatment, though in some cases other means of sperm retrieval may be needed.

For female patients one option is the collection of mature oocytes that can be used for IVF and subsequent embryo cryopreservation. The option of ovarian tissue harvesting is not always suitable for all patients but suggested criteria for the selection process have been drawn up by the Royal College of Obstetricians and Gynaecologists (Box 7.1).

The problem of assessing competence will be addressed in the next chapter, but we can see that fertility is a concern that adds an additional layer of anxiety for the young adult who not only has to absorb the fact that they have a life-threatening illness, but that even if they survive, they may be unable to have children. There are also gender differences that make the process more complex for girls and more embarrassing for boys. According to Dr Guy Makin, interviewed on the radio (*Woman's Hour* 2006), while cancer treatments may be less likely to result in infertility for girls, the harvesting of eggs is an invasive procedure that should not be undertaken lightly. In con-trast, while the collection of sperm is more straightforward, there are issues relating to the age of the young male. For example, it may not be easy to approach a 13-year-old boy and his family with the prospect of sperm col-lection, yet to fail to do so might have devastating consequences throughout that boy's life. As a result, Dr Makin suggested that boys as young as 13 should

Box 7.1 Edinburgh criteria for selection of patients for cryopreservation of ovarian cortical tissue

---

- Age < 30 years.

- No previous chemotherapy or radiotherapy (if aged < 15 years consider if previous 'low-risk' chemotherapy).

- A realistic chance of long-term survival.

- A high risk of treatment induced immediate ovarian failure (estimated at >50 per cent).

- Informed consent (from patient or, in the case of an incompetent child, from the parents).

- Negative HIV and hepatitis serology.

- No existing children.

Wallace and Brougham (2005: 145)

be offered advice on sperm banking, but as future fertility is unlikely to be a priority to boys of this age, it might be better offered as a routine treatment as boys (and their parents) may not request it.

The potential for embarrassment for boys is also great. Dan Jones, a teenager who had been through cancer said in the same interview, that his mother took him for his appointment to donate sperm and everyone knew exactly what he was doing while in the cubicle. Crawshaw (2006) reports that none of the participants in her research remembered having a choice about where the sample would be produced and collected, and those who were not given a choice about who would accompany them felt unsafe and un-supported. One suggestion for policy change that might address the embarrassment factor is for the collection process to be done at home rather than for the boy to have to be taken into a hospital environment. There are, however, issues relating to the viability of the sample so proximity to the laboratory freezing and storage facilities would have to be taken into account.

Perhaps surprisingly, according to Zebrack (2006: 227), there are reports that the prospect of infertility comes as a surprise to young adult cancer survivors who do not recall being told that their treatment might affect their future fertility. Thus it appears that in addition to professionals finding it difficult to discuss sexual matters (Shaw et al. 2004), there may be pockets of resistance to addressing the issue of fertility among staff who are not expert or trained in the field. According to Reebals et al. (2006), while 91 per cent of oncologists surveyed believed males undergoing chemotherapy *should* be offered sperm banking, 48 per cent either did not mention it or mentioned it to only 25 per cent of eligible males. Only 10 per cent claimed to have offered it to all eligible males.

Even if some of the lack of recall relates to the young person having forgotten rather than not having been informed, it would still appear that a more effective approach is needed so that the information can be retrieved at a later date when the young person is not in shock over the diagnosis and its implications.

The issues relating to fertility as raised by participants are discussed later in the chapter; however, we begin with the impact of the illness on establishing and maintaining sexual relationships.

The impact on sexual relationships

For those young people without partners at the time of diagnosis, there was the daunting prospect of having to tell a potential boyfriend or girlfriend about the illness and its possible legacy – both physical and emotional. However, the fear for many was that after the illness no one would be sexually attracted to them as the effect on their appearance would deter a potential partner. A number of the young people commented on the insecurities they now felt about their bodies and that this had undermined their belief that they would be found attractive. The prospect of meeting a new partner was intimidating, as is shown in the following quote from Philip. At the time of the interview he had what he hoped was a temporary colostomy after surgery for bowel cancer:

> I think if I had a permanent colostomy, I think, maybe that would have been different ... I mean, how do you bring it up first of all? Certainly having it at the moment I sometimes think, well if you meet someone and that, you go out with them a couple of times and think, when do I mention it? But once it goes, once I have my reversal, it's not going to be an issue, all I'll have is a scar and that's not a problem. They'll say, 'Oh, what did you get that from?' [I'll say] I had cancer and that's it, you know – job done ... I'm not quite as confident as I was, you know, I don't think I could chat to someone quite easily, you're always aware that it's there. All my friends say you'd never know which takes a lot of the pressure off but even so when you're sort of getting to know [someone] it's hard for a first time with people. It's just a barrier, well, you think it's a barrier really it doesn't need to be, you know.

> (Philip)

Philip had adopted an optimistic view of the future and envisaged a time when it would simply be a matter of explaining the scar, but in the meantime acknowledged that telling a potential girlfriend would be difficult. While Philip began by being quite positive, later in the quote he acknowledged that he could not 'chat to someone quite as easily' and that meeting people for the first time presented difficulties. The word 'barrier' is used twice, however, he rationalizes by saying that it doesn't need to be; nevertheless at an emotional level it seems that the prospect may still present problems for him. This extract conveys Philip's struggle in coming to terms with the albeit temporary physical effects of the illness.

Charlotte did not have a boyfriend at the time of her diagnosis and had held similar fears to Philip's that it would be difficult to find someone who would find her attractive. Yet, unexpectedly she started going out with her boyfriend after her illness had been diagnosed and while she was still in treatment:

> I met him after I'd lost my hair and everything, [he] really helped me with my confidence so that was good. I thought [boys] wouldn't be interested but it doesn't bother him, he just said, 'You know, it's just an illness, it's nothing to worry about.' So he doesn't mind.
>
> (Charlotte)

Charlotte's boyfriend lived round the corner, knew her well and had been aware of her illness before the relationship began, thus she had not been in the position of having to tell a relative stranger. She continued by saying what fun it was to be with her boyfriend and it was clear that his presence in her life at this stage when she could have been feeling unattractive and have feared that no one would be interested in her as a girlfriend had boosted her morale considerably.

Some of the young people were already in relationships before the illness. Nathan reflected on the effects his illness had had on several girlfriends:

> I'm nearly 18 and she's nearly 16, but she just wasn't grown up enough to ask questions and to know what I was going through and stuff. So that kind of didn't make me close to her ... I found her a bit ignorant about that.
>
> But I had [another] girlfriend ... and she was really good about it. But we just didn't see each other a lot so that's what kind of broke it up. And then I had [another] and she was just someone to be with ... that didn't work but hopefully when I get out of here and I get my hair back and my looks, hopefully I'll meet the right one.
>
> (Nathan)

In this case it seems that Nathan's first girlfriend had not had the maturity to deal with his illness, and though he does not specify why the next relationship broke up, the fact that they did not see each other much may have been related to the illness and Nathan's inability to undertake the usual social activities of the age group. We remember that Nathan had not wanted his friends to visit him in hospital because of his concern over his appearance. Thus it may have been that during his lengthy stays in hospital he discouraged visits from his girlfriends and this could have contributed to the short-lived nature of the relationships. It is also significant that Nathan hopes to meet 'the right one' when his hair has grown back and his 'looks' have been restored, these comments relate directly to issues about appearance and lack of confidence addressed in the previous chapter.

The eventual failure of a relationship was discussed by Michelle whose boyfriend had supported her through the acute stage of the illness and her treatment, but as she told me, the relationship had foundered subsequently:

> Actually, we only split up about three weeks ago ... we're still really good friends but that's all it had been, like, for a while, probably since I went into hospital. Because it's hard to keep things how they were. But he came to see me nearly every day ... visiting hours ... were two 'til eight and even if he didn't finish 'til eight o'clock, he'd always pop in for five minutes, when he'd finish work and stuff ... so, yes, he's helped me through it all. Like, I mean if anything else happens to me and I end up in hospital again for whatever reason, even though we're not together, I'd like my mum to tell him ... we still go out together and stuff ... I work with him as well so I see him at work.
>
> (Michelle)

It was unclear whether Michelle's relationship had come to an end because of the strain of the illness, but her comment that they were 'really good friends' and since her hospitalization that had been the basis of the relationship would strongly suggest that to be the case. At the time of the interview the break-up was recent and obviously still painful, thus it did not seem appropriate to press Michelle further to discuss how and why the relationship had failed. Nevertheless, from what she did say it appears that she valued her continued contact with her ex-boyfriend and she attributed no blame to him for them splitting up. So in this instance even though, unlike Nathan, Michelle was eager for her partner to visit her in hospital, this had not sustained the relationship in the longer term.

When she was diagnosed with ovarian cancer, Nicola and her partner had been expecting a baby that she had been advised to abort on medical grounds, thus, their relationship had been subject to considerable stress. In the lengthy quote that follows Nicola makes a number of points about how the illness affected her relationship. Some of these relate to her appearance and could have been included in the last chapter, and some relate to the difficult family dynamics, but the quote has been kept intact to maintain the power of its portrayal of the effect on her life:

> His mother actually died from the same cancer that I had. So he found it very, very hard, but saying that, he was very, very supportive. Especially about me losing my hair, because that was one thing I really, really didn't want to happen at all. And he took me to his guardian's house to get it shaved, and make it look reasonable. And he just had a laugh and a joke and just tried to make me feel as, as sexy as possible because I didn't feel like a woman anymore. I didn't feel right so he was very, very supportive, he still is actually ... unfortunately my partner doesn't get on with my father. So he would come down on a Saturday or a Sunday in the morning and he'd take me out for the day. Just locally and we'd sit in the car, and if I felt like I wanted to go for a walk he'd walk with me. And then we'd come back and we'd have dinner together as a family. And then he'd go about ten o'clock. So it was very difficult, I only actually saw him like once a week, but we spoke to each other every day obviously on the phone. And when I was in for my week of treatment I'd ring him up every night, about ten o'clock to let him know that I'd been unplugged from the chemo stand. So he'd sort of always giggle and I'd phone him up and he'd say 'Have you been unplugged?' I'm hanging out the window, 'Yes, I've been unplugged', which was great, it was hard but we got on with it.
>
> We did split up shortly after I had been given the all-clear. Because he later told me that he, every time he saw me, he thought of his mum. And that he hated me for the fact that I'd got better and his mother hadn't. So it was quite difficult to see that ... I understood completely ... I don't blame him in the slightest for feeling like that. But it was very, very hard for the few months that we had split up ... he just couldn't come to terms with it, and it's only recently that he's actually come to terms with the fact that I am here and it's tough basically ... [we were split up for] six months to a year ... but he was there for me while I was ill. And he was there for me when I needed him the most, although I felt that I needed him more for getting better and coping with going back to work, getting the hair, the daft things like that, and unfortunately he wasn't, but we did stay in touch. And I mean we've never been out of each other's lives for the past six years, even though we've been on and off. But we're back together now.
>
> (Nicola)

It is interesting that it was during her recovery that Nicola had felt the need for her boyfriend's presence, yet it might be assumed that the height of the illness is when the support is most needed. However, in the midst of the illness, life may be dominated by hospital stays, treatments and surgeries during which parents tend to take a key role. As Morgan and Hubber (2004) point out, a partner may only recently have 'joined' the family and thus may feel like an outsider who has no voice. Thus including a partner in such a scenario, particularly if as in this case he or she does not get on with the parents, may present challenges that the young person feels too ill to take on.

In a different context Steven reflected on the difficulties of his relationship with his partner Lisa's mother. The problem he encountered seems to have stemmed largely from her concerns about the impact his illness might have on her daughter's life:

> The cancer ... affected, not our relationship as such, but the relationship I had with her family ... Especially her mum ... don't get me wrong, I love them all to bits but it was quite odd at the time because they knew I had cancer obviously ... that all kind of worried her mum a bit. Lisa was never bothered really by it, but it worried her mum ... it was a 'What happens if he gets it again?' You know, but then it's, like, 'Well, then we'll deal with it if and when it happens' ... that took some sorting out really ... it was a bit awkward at times 'cause ... I always found it difficult to talk to her mum. Where her father, me and him got on ... like a house on fire straight away ... no problem ... we're good friends. But her mum, I had to sit down and talk to her like I'm talking to you now. It took conversation after conversation, hours after hours of explaining what I was doing ... You know – do I carry on with my life or do I just say sod it and give up? And that took some getting through to her; you know that took a bit of doing, did that.
>
> (Steven)

Yet Lisa and Steven's relationship had survived the impact of the illness and the reservations of Lisa's mother:

> She [Lisa] knows what'd happen if I got diagnosed again. You know, what I'd have to go through, what's expected of her as well. And she's good that way that she's just sort of accepted it as it is and if and when it does happen, then it happens and you know, we'll manage ... She helped a lot in the after effects. 'Cause like I say, I sort of went right off the idea of girls for probably a year or so ... it sounds selfish but all I was interested in was me. And when she sort of came onto the scene and we started dating and one thing and another and that

helped. It sort of felt more normal, more what I should have been doing. That was a nice change from 'You've got X amount of tablets to take on a morning; you've got to be here at this time of day for this treatment. You've got to be there at that time of day for that treatment, you've got to be . . .' ahh, your head just spun at times.

(Steven)

Clearly Steven's relationship with Lisa had been through some testing times, but having a girlfriend again after the illness and after having had no interest for 'a year or so' had, in his own words, made Steven feel more 'normal', he was now doing what a young man 'should be doing' after a life dominated by drug regimes and hospital appointments that, we remember from Chapter 5, were experienced by Steven as so frustrating, time-wasting and disruptive to normal life.

Gemma recounts the difficulty she had in telling her boyfriend, Dave, that she had cancer. She had already told her brother and sent a group text to her friends which she said she later regretted as a means to convey the news, but Dave who had rung her on his way home from Liverpool, she had not informed. Concerned that if she told him on the telephone he would be driving in a state of distress, she misled him and said that the results had not yet been given to her. However, she did tell him when he arrived home:

> Dave came home and I took him into the kitchen. He knew something was wrong and it felt like forever for my brain to try and tell him in the best way the result. But he just stood there with a look that I could not recognize – as if he was frozen. I needed him to hug me, have some sort of reaction, but he just stood there. I felt again that I had let him down. We had only been together for a year, he doesn't want a girlfriend with cancer.
>
> (Gemma)

Gemma's assumption was that after a relatively short time together her cancer would be experienced as a burden to Dave. However, from the remainder of Gemma's account, we can see that despite her concerns, her relationship with Dave survived the duration of her illness and he was able to offer her both emotional and financial support, though the relationship did not survive in the longer term.

> My theory is that if it, I didn't have the illness I think we would have actually broken up sooner. I didn't know whether he actually felt obliged to stay with me because I was ill rather than because he wanted to.
>
> (Gemma)

Marc said that he had 'a girlfriend at the time when I was poorly' but that the relationship had finished:

> It was a long-term one but I think it was just out of habit in the end. And then we finished just before I got ill. Then she was around because she felt guilty because I had [cancer] but we didn't want to be with each other, so we weren't going out with each other but we were just really good friends at the time, I think anyway. I don't know, it was quite a complicated situation then. But we're still friends now, better friends now than what we were.
>
> (Marc)

Here Marc too raised the issue of 'guilt' and duty, and felt that his girlfriend stayed with him out of a sense of obligation. This resonates with Gemma's account of her difficulty in telling her boyfriend as she did not want him to feel he had to support her out of duty and her subsequent suspicion that in fact he had done just that. In a relationship that may be at its outset, or not have the degree of commitment and stability that might be found in an older age group, knowing how or whether to stay together under such circumstances presents the young adults with considerable problems.

Even though Mark's marriage has survived the illness successfully, he had feared initially that his wife would stay with him out of pity:

> I was very scared and thought that she was stopping with me out of sympathy.
>
> You know for long periods of time I thought that ... if she did ever want to leave me that she wouldn't do ... because she felt sorry for me. Fortunately she said she never did, and she never left and we have a great relationship now.
>
> (Mark)

Being married, Mark arguably was in a more secure position, yet this did not appear to have allayed his fears; and it may be that the relationship has endured because of the commitment already made by getting married. While Emma and her partner Gary were still together, she said that the illness had resulted in tensions between them:

> Well, my boyfriend treats me differently ... we fall out all the time, we fell out loads of times since I found out because he doesn't understand that's why. Because he just doesn't understand, like he keeps telling me to shave my hair off and stuff like that. It's alright for him, because he's a man.
>
> (Emma)

Emma and Gary had two children, but in this age group many young people have not yet had children or made a commitment and thus the foundations of the relationship may be less secure. In a contrast to those young people who return to the parental home for care, thus undermining their relationship, the strain and tension that Dawn's illness caused between her parents resulted in her leaving the parental home where she had been living and as a consequence she moved in with her boyfriend. At the point when I spoke to her they had been living together for two years but she attributed the success of their relationship at least in part to her partner's age and maturity:

> I think the thing is that Paul is a bit older than me. He's nine years older than me, so he's 31, so he's quite mature. I think that, yes, if he'd been 20 as well, I think that might have been more difficult . . . I don't think we would have been together but he's older and he's got his own business and is quite mature. Well quite grown up, because men never grow up do they, apparently. But he's quite mature. He's got a business head on him.
>
> (Dawn)

Dawn continued by saying how supportive her partner had been and addressed the effect the illness had had on their sexual relationship:

> Because all this treatment affects your hormones . . . we are [sexually] active, aren't we . . . we're normal people [and] do want to have sex if you've got a partner . . . but you just don't feel like doing it . . . because you haven't got confidence, you just, I don't know what it is, it affects your hormones and you just don't have that sex hormone anymore . . . Paul, my partner wasn't bothered you know . . . take it or leave it . . . Like, most men, or girlfriends or whatever, might split up.
>
> (Dawn)

Dawn suspects that under the more usual circumstances of her partner being a similar age to her, their relationship may have failed, indicating that age and consequently life stage are crucial. Again we see the issue of lack of confidence raised, echoing many comments in the last chapter. It is of course likely that cancer in other age groups affects levels of self-confidence and libido, yet for an older and more firmly established couple the insecurity might not be felt so acutely. This is borne out by Kelly's account. We remember from the previous chapter that she was extremely distressed about her weight gain, yet when she talked about how it had affected her relationship with her husband, it was clear that she had no insecurities or anxieties about his reaction:

He's been absolutely fantastic. He really has been so supportive and he's never [said] 'Oh, look at all this weight' and he's, like, 'Well, don't worry about it you'll lose it all you know.' He's been brilliant, nothing's changed really . . . Yes, but he's been absolutely fantastic . . . [he] doesn't complain at all.

(Kelly)

Again this quote suggests that the stability of a more mature relationship, marriage and children lends security to the situation that is missing for those at the younger end of the age range. Ross and his partner Hannah may not have been married but were living together when Ross was diagnosed at the age of 23. They both agreed that their relationship had been strengthened:

I think it's made us stronger hasn't it? You know, our bond is stronger.

(Ross)

We're very close now, aren't we?

(Hannah)

Yes. You know because we've been through so much together, a lot more than most people have been through. So I think it brings you closer then.

(Ross)

However, we remember from the last chapter that they had been fortunate enough to be able to sustain their independence and remain living together, again indicating that the more established the relationship at the point of diagnosis, the greater the likelihood of its survival. While such an observation might seem self-evident, relationships in this age group and at this life stage are frequently newly formed and fragile and are thus disproportionately affected by life-threatening illness (Grinyer 2002a).

Fertility

Because of the age group and life stage of the participants, the likelihood of already having parented a child or completed a family may be remote, yet many young adults with cancer will be facing treatment that could compromise their future fertility. The majority of the participants had not already had children, only Kelly and Emma were mothers at the time of their diagnoses, and we remember that Nicola had needed to have an abortion as she was pregnant when diagnosed.

Despite having had ovarian cancer and a medical termination, at the time of the interview Nicola was six months pregnant and had become pregnant without any medical intervention. Since the interview she has given birth to a healthy baby. However, here she reflects on her reaction when at 13 weeks pregnant she was told the first pregnancy was unviable and also that she might become infertile:

> I was told that a termination had to be done because obviously the treatment wouldn't let a child survive . . . and obviously my fertility was a big issue to me . . . So we came up with all these questions, and my partner came with me, not my mum. I wanted him to be there because I'd asked my mum what . . . questions she felt I should ask, because obviously you're not in the right state of mind after hearing something as horrendous as that. So we asked the questions, I asked about the fertility and they said that obviously there is a chance that you may not [be fertile after treatment] but because you need to be treated as quickly as possible there's no chance that we can save any eggs or anything like that. Which I was absolutely mortified about, absolutely horrified. And I was storming round saying 'If I was a bloke I would, it wouldn't be the same . . .'
>
> (Nicola)

The decision to agree to an abortion was not one taken lightly by Nicola but her boyfriend, the baby's father, was unwilling to lose them both, thus helping her to reach her decision:

> I sort of almost went into a world of my own . . . my partner . . . said to me that . . . basically that if I don't get the treatment and done, and have the termination done, he would have to deal with two deaths and he can't deal with that. He can only just deal with the idea of losing the baby but not me as well. So that sort made me think, right, well, Ok, I'll do it, I'm young enough to get over it. And I'm young enough to sort of fight as much as I can, and all I can do is try.
>
> (Nicola)

The anger represented in Nicola's words 'storming around' is echoed in the following account from Gemma who shouted every swear word she could think of, but in this case in her head rather than aloud:

> Because of my age and that it had most likely been caught early, I had a good prognosis. I would have to go through chemotherapy and radiotherapy. I didn't take in everything, just stared at him trying to think of questions, the first thing was about my fertility. I've just

been told I have cancer and I'm worried about having kids, why did I ask that? It seemed so trivial looking back; surely there were more important questions I should have asked? I was shouting every swear word I could think of in my head. I repeated back what he had told me to get it straight.

(Gemma)

It is interesting that Gemma should have felt that in retrospect a question about fertility was relatively trivial, while she may not have had the anguish that Nicola was subject to over her decision to abort, Gemma was nevertheless facing a future of possible infertility. However, the distress of infertility is not felt only by young women. Even though Nicola's assumption was that had she 'been a bloke' the problem would not have been as great, Nathan, a down-to-earth young man undertaking a joinery apprenticeship, showed considerable emotion when he recollected the only experience of his cancer journey that had reduced him to tears:

I knew it was cancer and stuff but I never knew anyone with cancer so I wasn't really bothered about it. And then I saw my consultant and he told me about all the treatment and the only time that I cried was when he said I might not be able to have kids like [in the] proper way. So that got me upset but I did some banking for that.

(Nathan)

It appears that Nathan had previously been unaware that cancer treatment could result in infertility, but he was at least able to bank sperm. He spoke of his hopes of meeting 'the right girl' and that she would understand the situation and that at some stage in the future he could father children even if, as he put it, it was not 'in the proper way'. The fact that Nathan used such a phrase suggests that the possible future need for artificial insemination continued to cause him some distress. Mark, already married and 'trying for a family' before he was diagnosed, told me that his wife had undergone a miscarriage 18 months before his diagnosis with testicular cancer, thus the prospect of infertility had caused great concern to them both and Mark had banked sperm as a precaution. However, he had subsequently fathered two children naturally and had the banked sperm destroyed.

In contrast, Steven was relatively sanguine about the prospect; he was in a stable relationship and in the process of setting up home with his partner Lisa. In relationship to fertility, he said the following:

She [Lisa] knows the chances are we might not be able to have kids . . . we never really talked about it. It was not that it was a forbidden subject, but it never sort of came up. You know, nobody ever questioned it ... [I] know that I might not be able to have kids; there is a small chance that I can't. And I've never been tested after the treatment to say whether I can or not ... don't get me wrong, I do think about it, and I often [wonder] shall I just get tested but at the minute we're not bothered, we're not actually looking for kids, and you know we're more worried about the house, what wallpaper ... what door do we buy? Well, that's about our biggest worry at the minute you know, what car am I buying next? And that's the way we like it at the minute ... we don't plan really ... I don't know whether that's part of the cancer ... because another friend of mine, he's settled down now. He's actually married and he's got a kid on the way ... he seems to have his job organized and he knows what he wants to do and, me, I don't know what I want to do tomorrow. I don't know what I want for my tea when I leave here. You know, I haven't got a clue. And to be quite honest I'm quite happy living like that.

(Steven)

It appears that Steven's illness has resulted in him 'living for the day', making the most of every opportunity to be spontaneous and apparently not wishing, at least at this stage, to be tied down by children. Ross was similarly sanguine about his probable infertility and appeared more concerned about the implications for his partner Hannah:

There's a good chance I could be sterile so I've got some sperm frozen in the sperm bank for the future ... it doesn't upset me or bother me really ... as long as I'm alright, I'm not bothered ... there's more important things than that. I suppose it's a bigger issue for Hannah than me now, because if we do have to use it, I don't have to do anything, it's Hannah that has to go through the ordeal of having artificial insemination ... Actually, children is just not an issue with us at the moment, you know, because Hannah has to finish Uni and then get married and then I suppose children ... providing everything's still going alright. So it could be, I don't know, five years away yet. But [to Hannah] I don't think you'll be looking forward to it will you?

(Ross)

These accounts contrast sharply with Nathan's grief at his probable inability to father children naturally with a partner he had not even met. Perhaps this is because he was concerned that not already being in a relationship, his possible infertility might make it less likely that he would meet a partner who accepted the situation, while Steven was already secure in his relationship with Lisa and Ross with Hannah. This may be endorsed by Philip's account of his probable infertility and the fact that it had been his girlfriend who accompanied him to donate sperm:

> Before I had my first dose of chemo they sent me down to Manchester to leave a sample and stuff, they say, after the chemo, I can go back and be tested to see whether I am [fertile], whether I do or not we'll see. I can quite honestly say at the moment I'm not bothered about having kids at all, it probably won't bother me until I want kids . . . it was quite hard giving the sample, you know, doing it under pressure and things like that . . . I went on my own first time, then second time [my] girlfriend came down with me because I had to do it a second time. Because of that I probably won't bother going there again. If I ever want a child I'll try and try and if it doesn't happen it's obvious why.
>
> (Philip)

What this account raises is the difficulty of donating sperm – not a topic that is easy to address. Most young men and their peers might assume that sperm banking, while stressful, is at least relatively straightforward, but of course the very reason for its need is that the young man is extremely ill and also by definition it is done under pressure, as Philip acknowledges. Marc also intimated that sperm donation had not been without its challenges, in his case because he was recovering from surgery at the time:

> It was a long time between my operation getting transferred to the clinic so I wasn't too well, and then it was all rushed . . . I did give my donation [but] it wasn't very good because I'd just had my operation so . . . it could have been better . . . you can go for a check and it's nice to know where you stand.
>
> (Marc)

Despite saying that it would have been nice to know where he stood, meaning that he would like to know whether or not he was fertile, Marc went on to say that as he was not currently in a relationship, he was not really that worried about it. This contrasts with Nathan's fears for a future relationship in which infertility might be a problem.

In Chapter 4 we saw accounts of negotiating independence from parents that extend to medical consultations and encounters and clearly being accompanied to the hospital by his mother is likely to be stressful for a young man when donating sperm. The need to undertake such a challenge without being accompanied by his mother was addressed by Steven:

> I never refused my mum and dad, well, only once I refused my mum to go to the hospital and that was when I went to St Mary's for my

semen sample. That was a bit embarrassing, so she didn't come. My dad took me down, because he knew where the hospital was as it happened ... And that wasn't a problem, but I couldn't have my mum go to that one. That was the only time that she didn't go to the hospital with me ... it was my mum who used to take me down ... every day because my dad ... works shifts. ... Lisa [Steven's partner] goes in with me. And you know, like, we have, you know, we have no secrets about what goes on ... she knows what I've been through.

(Steven)

Clearly for a young man to be accompanied by his mother on a visit to donate sperm presents potential difficulties (Crawshaw 2006). This was acknowledged in the interview with Dr Makin on *Woman's Hour* (2006) who suggested the provision of home visits might make the situation easier for the young men. In this case it might have alleviated some of the embarrassment if a time had been arranged when Steven could have had the house to himself and not been reliant on his mother or father for transport to hospital.

Kelly knew that her fertility might have been compromised by her illness and treatment, and was profoundly thankful that she had already had a child before her diagnosis:

Well, they said initially there's a 20 per cent chance that, you know, I might not be able to have children. And me and John, we sort of discussed it, you know. At the end of the day we're very lucky to have one so it's just one of them things, you know, if we try for one and it happens, it happens. If it doesn't ... if I hadn't had any children, I think I would have been in quite a turmoil now. I went to see a nurse down at the Unit ... she gave me a phone number to ring, to some specialist in London who deals with fertility in cancer. And she says, you know, give her a ring if you want to. But the thing was, when she actually rang me with this number, it was the night before I was to start treatment and I would have had to delay treatment and you know it was like, 'Oh, what do I do, what do I do?' And I just wanted to get on with it, really. You know, I'd just had enough of waiting because I think it was about two months from being diagnosed to starting treatment.

(Kelly)

Kelly had already waited five months for the diagnosis and then another two before starting treatment, the prospect of further delay while she went through egg harvesting was clearly not acceptable to her, yet as she acknowledged, she might have felt very differently if she and her husband had not already had a child. There was also the issue of travelling to London (from the north of England) for treatment and the prospect of a lengthy trip was not something she could face, yet it appeared that no local provision for the more complex procedure of egg collection had been offered to her.

Discussion

We begin by returning to the issue of forming or sustaining a relationship after diagnosis and treatment. It is clear from the accounts above that the difficulties experienced in terms of self-confidence build on the issues discussed in the last chapter to undermine the young people's belief that they will be found sexually attractive and be able to make new relationships. This is exacerbated by age and life stage as it is at this point in their lives and development that young people pay a great deal of attention to physical appearance (Hain 2005; Lewis 2005) and the forming of sexual relationships (Craig 2006).

Most of the young people in the study were in relationships at the time of diagnosis and some of these had survived despite the stress of the illness. Others had found that their relationship could not withstand the demands and effects of the illness or feared that a partner was only staying with them out of a sense of duty. For these young people, having to let go of the relationship as well as facing an uncertain future proved challenging. For those who hoped to establish a relationship at a later stage, the prospect appeared daunting. This is redolent of George's fears when on an early visit to the oncologist George asked his father the question, 'Will anybody ever love me with a metal knee?' (Grinyer 2002a: 68).

The forming of new sexual relationships among teenagers and young adults is perhaps a more central part of their life stage than at any other period. The anxieties that are provoked by insecurities about body image and attractiveness have been expressed by many of the young people and summed up in George's comment above. Yet if Shaw et al. (2004) are right, many nurses are ill prepared to engage with and support their young patients in this area, but, as these authors say, with appropriate training, they would be in a pivotal position to assist the adolescent cancer patient – again suggesting that it is in the specialist care setting that staff are more likely to develop expertise and learn strategies to feel comfortable in addressing this important issue.

We saw from Kelly's example of being slightly older and having moved through the transition into the next stage of life, the infrastructure of her life and the stability of her marriage ameliorated some of the insecurities felt by those at the younger end of the age range. In the last chapter we saw that she was as concerned about her appearance as any other participant, but at least she had a firm belief in her husband's commitment to her and that any physical changes were understood and accepted by him. The same applies to her perspective on fertility, having already had a child at the point of diagnosis, some of the issues relating to the risk of future sterility were mitigated.

The prospect of not having further children may have been a source of regret but not the tragedy it would have been had she not had a pre-existing child. Indeed, many of the other participants expressed considerable anger at the prospect that they may remain childless.

A central theme of this volume is the concept of young adulthood, but as we have seen, there are many life stages along the continuum that raise questions about the similarity of experience, for example, between a 14-year-old and a 24-year-old. Yet the prospect of future infertility for a cohort that is largely childless is an issue that binds together the age range across the spectrum and crosses the gender divide. There are, of course, options for the preservation of future fertility and while these may be technically more straightforward for young men, the prospect of emotional distress and embarrassment still need to be addressed, while for the young women the time-consuming and invasive nature of the procedure must be considered. We saw at the start of the chapter that in theory the cryopreservation of eggs for later usage or for IVF treatment and embryo cryopreservation is a possibility for young women. Yet it is clear from Nicola's account that her urgent need for treatment may render such an option unviable in that it could cause a dangerous delay, or, as in Kelly's case, apparently treatment may be unavailable through local provision.

It is also the case that in order for IVF treatment to take place at the time of egg harvesting, the young woman would need to have a partner to fertilize the eggs, and it is perhaps less likely that at this life stage a lasting relationship will have been established. Even a partner able and willing to provide sperm might at a later point, if the relationship failed, withdraw consent for the implantation of a fertilized egg. The high profile court case taken by Natalie Evans demonstrates the potential legal risks relating to such a procedure. In Ms Evans' case, embryos had been created prior to cancer treatment that was certain to lead to her infertility as she had both ovaries removed. However, her ex-fiancé whose sperm had been used to fertilize the eggs when they were a couple, refused his consent for implantation after his relationship with Ms Evans failed, despite the cryopreservation of the embryos stored on the assumption they would be implanted after her recovery (*Guardian*, 8 March 2006: 5). Ms Evans lost her case at the High Court and subsequently at the Court of Appeal. Following this, the judgment of the Strasbourg Court also found against her right for implantation to proceed. The stress endured indicates that the option of IVF and the cryopreservation of embryos can be fraught with potential long-term risks. Ms Evans was in her early thirties when diagnosed with cancer yet the chance that a relationship between significantly younger partners may not survive seems even greater. As we have seen, the stress the illness causes to relationships, particularly at the younger end of the age range, may result in their longer-term failure and a possible legal wrangle over the right to implant embryos.

The centrality of these issues and their potential to cause distress and the consequent danger of non-compliance indicate that expertise needs to be developed among staff who are trained to support both young men and young women through the decision-making processes while offering them the best chance for future procreation. The implications for policy and practice are addressed in greater detail in the final chapter.

Key points

Effects on sexuality are far-reaching because:

- relationships may be fragile;

- relationships may be unstable;

- relationships may not yet have been formed;

- fear of partner staying out of duty;

- self-confidence eroded;

- lack of libido;

- embarrassment;

- disclosure difficult;

- partner may not understand.

Fertility issues are particularly problematic because:

- infertility can result before children have been conceived;

- families not yet completed;

- sperm donation embarrassing;

- sperm donation difficult;

- sexual maturity needed for sperm donation;

- egg harvesting invasive;

- partner required for embryo cryopreservation;

- pregnancy may need to be terminated;

- treatment causing infertility may be refused.

---

8 The implications for policy and practice

Defining the characteristics of the age group: the relationship to care

This volume began by asking whether teenagers and young adults, who encompass such a wide range of life styles and experiences, could be defined as a distinct group. The testimonies of the participants suggest strongly that this is the case. The issues raised by the participants were those of importance to them rather than being predetermined by research questions and these issues have fitted into a themed organization under chapter headings. This implies a commonality of experience that, while not generalizable, indicates that life stage has shaped the experience in similar ways for the participants.

Despite the age range having been wide and having encompassed a variety of life styles and experiences, there are factors that unite the group. However, within the upper age range of the participants, it was possible to discern the beginnings of a change in the weighting and emphasis of some of the issues. Indeed, it would have been surprising had this not been the case, as this is a transitional period of great change. Nevertheless, even without the reification of life stage and the drawing of firm boundaries around it, there still appears to be compelling evidence that those in the age range require the provision of specialist services. One factor that unites them is their lack of an easy fit within a system that may fail to accommodate their needs, physical, social and emotional, outside of the specialist setting of care.

In the preceding chapters there were examples of insensitive or even bad practice that would be experienced as distressing and unacceptable by any patient at whatever age – in which case, we might ask the question 'Why is it any worse for this age group?' However, a young person who is subjected to bad practice may not have the life experience that would allow him or her to manage the encounter with confidence or to see it in perspective. They may also be unwilling to let parents intercede on their behalf while they struggle to retain fading vestiges of independence.

Kelly, the oldest participant at 26, married and with a child at the point of diagnosis, shared many of the same concerns as younger participants. She felt marginalized in a non-age-specific setting of care and she had endured a lengthy period of delay before an accurate diagnosis was made in circumstances that suggest her age was a factor. She was also very distressed about her change in appearance, particularly the weight gain that troubled the younger cancer patients. These similarities suggest that at the upper end of the age range there is a period of transition whereby some but not all of the life stage issues are still experienced. The instances where her perspective differed also help to illuminate specific life stage issues. Kelly's stability, security and previously well-established independence meant that her need for renewed dependence on her parents was not experienced as threatening. Her relationship with her husband precluded the insecurity and anxiety about the prospect of developing a new sexual relationship in the future, and the fact that she already had a child lessened her distress at the prospect of future infertility.

The professionals' perspective

Most of the professionals in the age-specific care settings also had experience of providing care to other age groups and were as a result able to offer a degree of comparison by identifying characteristics that differentiated young adulthood. The professionals working outside the age-specific setting were able to reflect on the management of the situation without specialist expertise. This range of professional experience may help to illuminate not only best practice in the specialist care setting, but also help us to understand the barriers and problems facing professionals in the non-specialist setting.

So what defining characteristics do professionals identify in the age group? Discussions with a range of specialist health care and support staff indicated that those in the age group are united by a key feature, which is a burning desire for their individuality to be recognized explicitly and a need to be 'treated like normal teenagers'; their identity outside the setting of care taking precedence over that of their identity as a patient. As Deborah, staff nurse on the TCT ward, put it: 'Their needs predominantly are to be individuals ... they just want to be treated as normal teenagers who have got an illness of some description, rather than defined by the fact that they have got cancer.'

The focus on the need to be treated primarily as an individual was implicit in much of the participants' interview data and the significance of acknowledging an identity that transcended that of 'cancer patient' was clear. While this might represent good practice at any age, and indeed for any illness, in previous research (Grinyer 2002a), it became apparent that teenagers and young adults are at a transitional stage when childhood identity is being left behind, and adult identity has yet to be formed fully. As a result, the loss of a fragile and insecure identity may be experienced by young adults as particularly undermining. It also seems that the additional shock of the diagnosis being 'cancer' sets these young people apart from those who live with other congenital, chronic and life-limiting illnesses.

Managing the needs of young adults

Attempts at maintaining their easily broken hold on independence and identity can result in behaviour that may be deemed unwise and challenging by professionals and parents (Grinyer 2002a). Indeed, it became clear from discussions with some professionals in practice outside the specialist centres that they found it difficult to treat the young people who were perceived as impatient and demanding. I heard reports of young adults being described as 'awkward' and difficult to manage. Yet no criticisms of the young adults' attitudes or behaviour were made in the age-specific care settings which raises the question of whether their behaviour in the specialist setting was 'better' as a result of feeling less alienated, or whether the staff in the specialist environment were more practised at managing manifestations of anxiety and distress. Sue, Lead Macmillan Clinical Nurse Specialist for teenagers and young adults states:

> Many of them won't say 'thank you' – but, that's not why we are here. They aren't in the least bit demanding – challenging, yes, demanding – no! I don't think that they go out to please you, but they will challenge you – they will soon know if you are telling an untruth. Many of them are compliant – often because they don't think that they have a choice – they are too scared to not do as we say – but, that in itself isn't very healthy. They need to know that they have a voice and a certain amount of choice in what happens to them – if they are quiet and compliant, I would worry – you need that spark.
>
> (Sue)

Yet even when challenging behaviour is exhibited, this is accompanied by vulnerability, while young adults can be fiercely independent one day, they can manifest an almost childlike dependence the next. This paradox relates as well to the apparent contradiction between being challenging and compliant.

> It is in this age group that we get non-compliance – young people who think that they can refuse treatment, for example – because they think that they are immortal, or because they are terrified of the whole process. This takes a lot of skill and team working, and by team I mean that we include the young people and their families. This is why we need skilled professionals to care for them.
>
> (Sue)

So we can see many contradictions, the young adults can be compliant and non-compliant, challenging and acquiescent, independent and vulnerable.

These apparent paradoxes are characteristic of an age group that is itself transitional, fluid and changing. All these issues are being fought out under 'normal' circumstances and thrown into sharp relief under duress. As Craig (2006: 117) argues, 'it is important that staff are aware of the difficulties faced in "normal" adolescence ...' in order that they can understand and best support the young person and their family during this time of additional stress, and it is likely that it will be in the specialist setting that such expertise can be developed across the care team.

Supporting a social network

Also of fundamental importance at this insecure stage of life is the need to belong, to be accepted by a peer group and to share an identity with them while – again paradoxically – also establishing individuality and in- dependence. However, while friends and a peer group may be of central im- portance, separation from them is likely because, as we saw in Chapter 3, there can be reluctance on the part of the young adults to allow them to visit, and friends can be unwilling to visit. Additionally in Chapter 5, we saw that friends are moving on through the transitional life stage themselves and may thus become geographically distant and unavailable. In any case, contact will be limited by the need to withdraw from school or college, thus social iso- lation is a real danger for a number of different reasons. Craig (2006) points out that young people attach great importance to being part of a social scene.

The importance of the mutuality, supportive environment and sense of belonging offered by a support group either professionally or peer led, has been established by Ussher et al. (2006). Yet, as Zebrack (2006: 231) says, this is an opportunity rarely offered to adolescents and young adults with cancer. Thus the presence of a peer group in the care setting can fulfil this function and mitigate the isolation experienced when treated in a non-specialist en- vironment as the only young adult with cancer. As Geehan, herself a young adult cancer patient says: 'being "in the same boat" is very special and pro- cures a real sense of family' (2003: 2682).

Improving outcomes

Improving diagnosis

The material upon which Chapter 2 is based suggests that there is a lack of early recognition and diagnosis that may lead to the cancer being detected at a later stage of the disease when it has become less treatable. The delays, as we have seen, originate in both medical staff and the young patients. Staff in the specialist centres were well aware of delayed diagnosis as a problem and the accounts presented here act to support the strong suspicions of those such as

Lewis (2005) and Whiteson (2005) who have suggested that more evidence is needed on such delays. But the crucial question remains, what can be done to speed up the process so that symptoms are presented earlier and dealt with more quickly?

Dr James, in his capacity as a GP in a university practice and thus working predominantly among young people, suggested that a characteristic of the age group is to 'bury their heads in the sand and hope it will go away'. To address this tendency, he recommended the provision of information that targeted specific cancers associated with young adulthood. He used the example of an educational campaign among first year university students, alerting them to the dangers of testicular cancer. Leaflets were handed out to both male and female students and the result was a rise in presentations, referrals and early treatments of actual cancers. It is arguable that to focus on the cancers that are most prevalent among young adults in the places where young adults are concentrated such as schools, colleges, universities, and new recruits in the armed services would have the effect, not only of educating the young person, but also of heightening the awareness of primary care health workers.

The chances of early identification would be increased if doctors were trained to be alert to the possibility of cancer as a diagnosis in young adults through a formal training agenda. However, Michelagnoli et al. (2003: 2571) argue that the discipline of 'Adolescent Medicine', which might incorporate the necessary clinical acumen, is not taught uniformly across the world. These authors propose that such training might in addition incorporate non-traditional – and more appropriate – means of patient–professional communication including websites, e-mail and text messaging. It could also be argued that increased recognition within health service provision that young adulthood merits specialist cancer care settings could act to alert those within the medical professions – and the public – that cancer does indeed affect this age group and should be considered as a possibility and investigated at an early stage.

In addition, the testimony of other young adults who have had cancer could contribute to raising awareness. In Chapter 2 we saw that Mark's acquaintance had only sought medical advice for his testicular cancer because he had known about Mark's illness. As a result, Mark suggested that he would like to take part in an awareness raising campaign in schools to alert young people to the dangers, yet he was afraid that if he 'went public' in this way, his daughters would be teased by children taunting them with 'your dad's only got one ball', that he said was 'the only thing that really does hold me back'. This is a pity as he and other survivors might have much to offer, personal experience being a powerful way to communicate health-related information.

Improving compliance

One of the aims of the research has been about 'improving experience', and this cannot be separated from 'improving outcomes' as the two are inextricably and, I would argue, causally linked particularly in relationship to achieving compliance. In a note in Chapter 1 I suggested that a more appropriate descriptor for 'compliance' might be 'therapeutic convergence' as it implies a collaborative relationship between patients and those involved in their care, and this appears to be fundamental to the philosophy in the specialist units where staff engage in a partnership with the young adults. Indeed, it was clear in Emma's case that her eventual 'compliance' was achieved solely through being referred to a specialist unit.[1]

As Albritton and Bleyer (2003: 2595) document, the age group are associated with non-compliance in a range of other chronic diseases such as HIV, and Haase (2004: 289) claims that 'adolescents frequently demonstrate a lack of commitment to following treatment protocols'. Indeed, Thomas et al. (2006) claim that this age group demonstrates a particularly high incidence of poor adherence which has been reported to be as high as 59 per cent.

If non-compliance is in fact this high, the importance of the psychosocial challenges being understood and managed supportively is crucial and is more likely among specialist staff who develop the kind of expertise that may increase the likelihood of compliance and thus ultimately survival rates. The wide range of support – medical, psychological, social, and practical – required to maximize compliance is best provided by a multidisciplinary team approach[2] and this is again more likely to be found in the specialist centres. Haase and Phillips (2004: 146) point out that the young adults tend to construct their own view of illness and treatment that influences their commitment to adherence, thus interventions that are not grounded in their experiences are unlikely to be effective.

Clinical trials

There is an argument that systematically organized care for the age group may ultimately lead to better medical outcomes and increase survival rates. According to Lewis (2005: 253), the centralization of care improves outcomes especially in the case of rare tumours and those requiring complex treatment and this may also reduce physical late effects. Given that Bleyer et al. claim that in addition to the particular psychological and social needs of young adults with cancer, the 'spectrum of malignant diseases is different from that in any other period in life' (2005: 43), it is important that the specific characteristics of disease in adolescence are understood and managed in a more structured, systematic and coherent fashion by standardizing treatments according to agreed protocols based on inclusion in clinical trials. Even the cancers that are found in other age groups have a different aetiology in young adulthood. As Thomas et al. say, 'morphologically similar cancers may be molecularly distinct in ways that basic and clinical research may resolve' (2006: 303). And according to Albritton and Bleyer (2003), there will need to be an adjustment to therapy that has been formulated for either children or older adults whose tumours may have a different biology. Yet if those in the age group are scattered across a variety of treatment centres, it is likely that this will present barriers to research as only a few institutions can develop clinical expertise or take part in clinical trials.

Lewis argues that there is evidence that patients entered into clinical trials have better outcomes; yet as Bleyer et al. (2005) demonstrate, young adults with cancer are less likely than either children or older adults to be included in a clinical trial. Michelagnoli et al. (2003) claim in striking contrast to children under 14, 90 per cent of whom are entered into at least one clinical trial, the figure for those from 14–29 can be as low as 36 per cent. However, according to Michelagnoli et al., the likelihood of inclusion in clinical trials increases with specialist provision: 'With proper referral patterns to adolescent Units equipped with data managers and with strong links to national and international collaborative trial groups the figure for the younger people should rise' (2003: 2572). The improvement in outcomes associated with clinical trials, coupled with the likelihood that such trials will lead to a better understanding of the particular biological characteristics of adolescent cancers, provides yet another imperative for the development of specialist treatment centres.

The role of the family and managing consent

A thread that runs throughout this volume and the testimonies of the young people is the importance of families. While on occasion there has been a comment that suggests a mother may have been perceived as overly anxious or protective, implicitly throughout the accounts is evidence that family support is fundamental. It may be tacit and taken for granted, nevertheless, the role of family appears to be crucial.

While I was collecting data on the specialist ward, a parent, usually the mother, but also on occasions a father or other relative, was with the patient. They were often at the bedside or in the day room with their son or daughter; rarely it seems socializing with each other, though if they were making a drink or getting something to eat at the same time in the day room, they would exchange pleasantries. Thus families were a characteristic and ever present feature of the specialist ward. As Morgan and Hubber (2004: 130) say, 'cancer in adolescence causes exceptional stress in the family' and in re-cognition of this a philosophy of 'family-centred care' has been adopted in the specialist care setting that offers support to the families, carers and close friends.

From the patient's perspective, Geehan, diagnosed at 17, reflects on the role her family were encouraged to take in the age-specific setting where her osteosarcoma was treated:

> Parents are actively encouraged to get involved and participate ... in their children's treatment. This helps to reduce the wretched feelings of helplessness they might experience if they just have to sit and watch ... with the greater understanding they acquire they become a hugely important source of support to their children. This ... helps the patients develop a crucial trust in the abilities of their parents to look after them confidently when they go home.
>
> (Geehan 2003: 2682)

Yet managing the family's role may on occasion prove challenging for professionals caring for this age group which, as Bearison (2006) says, can create enormous problems for staff. Parents may still be adjusting to taking a more passive role and relinquishing responsibility for their son's or daughter's health care. This changing dynamic can be difficult for the parents and requires the need for careful management by professionals who, it seems, according to Geehan (2003,) are skilfully and appropriately included in the care of their sons and daughters.

While acknowledging the importance of their involvement and support, families can manifest over-protectiveness; this issue was raised by Diane, the sister on the TCT ward: 'The young person is quite independent ... [they] need the family around but not necessarily as much as that family want ... they're not wanting to take the family back on board as much as the family wants to be involved.'

Young adults not treated in the specialist environment are also likely to have families with them for much of the time, and of course they are in close attendance in the family home where community-based care and recovery are most likely to take place. Some of the professionals outside the specialist setting indicated that dealing with the family's involvement could be problematic, but in the specialist care setting the potential for conflict was recognized as a normal part of the process, handled with skill by experienced staff and perhaps pre-empted by their carefully managed inclusion (Geehan 2003).

Despite the possibility of tensions, discussions with professionals in the specialist setting indicated recognition that families provide a vital support structure for their sons and daughters. Thus the provision of accommodation on the hospital premises or financial assistance for other accommodation was acknowledged as an important feature of the wider care package. Given their pivotal role, this means that the recognition of parents' fears and changing relationship with their son or daughter has to be accommodated by professionals.

The families of young adults are also likely to want a role in decision-making and to be present when information is given, though, as Morgan and Hubber (2004) point out, many parents struggle with the fact that their son or daughter may want to be in control of their treatment decisions. As Lewis (2005) says, for this age group participation and a level of control in decision-making that leads to patients being able to make choices are important. This is the approach taken by Morgan and Hubber:

> Literature has identified that coping and compliance with treatment improve when patients feel that they are in control of a situation. These young people have been encouraged, with much guidance from professionals, to lead in their cancer journey, and by giving them access to information and peer support they are able to feel in control.
>
> (2004: 137)

Parents need support and reassurance through the process of relinquishing control and a key role of the nurse is to help to facilitate partnerships between the different parties. In some cases, according to Morgan and Hubber, this involves 'being an advocate for all members of the group surrounding the patient in order to achieve support and appropriate control for all parties' (2004: 130). Lewis and Morgan, both from a specialist setting and expert in managing such a scenario, acknowledge that parents can find the process challenging:

> As children approach adulthood their involvement in the consent process increases significantly. The idea that children and young people should receive information about cancer, and be involved in giving consent, can be disturbing for parents struggling to come to terms themselves and who naturally wish to protect their child.
>
> (2006: 6)

Lewis and Morgan explain the process of the giving and sharing of information and decision-making (2006: 6). Children older than 11 are usually given more detailed information than those younger than 11 and this will normally be shared with their parents at the same time, provided all are agreed on this course of action. There is an emphasis on ensuring that the young adult understands the full implications of the proposed treatment regime. Lewis and Morgan say that in the majority of cases there is full agreement between the parents, their son or daughter and the health professionals.

If this is the case, they are all asked to sign a consent form so that treatment can proceed. Even those patients under the age of 16 are encouraged to countersign the form, despite the legal consent having been provided by the parent or guardian. This means that they have been involved fully in the process. Lewis and Morgan provide a checklist for assessing competence (Box 8.1).

Box 8.1 Competence assessment checklist

• They understand what the treatment is and why they require it.
• They understand the benefits, risks and any alternatives.
• They understand what will happen if they don't have the treatment.
• They understand the information long enough to make a decision.
• They can make a choice.

(Lewis and Morgan 2006: 7)

However clear these guidelines are, conflict may arise involving decisions around end of life care and when treatment should make way for palliative care. According to George and Hutton: 'The natural causal consequence is for us all to seek increasingly futile solutions ... in such situations we create a climate of denial and frenetic "last ditches" that leave us all when facing death feeling hopeless, helpless and guilty' (2003: 2663).

In Deborah's experience, a young person might accept that the time had come to relinquish the 'frenetic last ditches' to refuse treatment and to 'let go', but this was never acceptable to the parents:

> The parents that I've come across without exception just wanted to fight. It was very, very difficult [for them] to accept the potential loss of the child ... that potentially would be a conflict area ... palliative and terminal treatment [is] bound to be a difficult issue ... for a [young person] who's going through this their feelings probably would be 'This is what I've done, this is where I've been and this is enough for me. I'm ready now, I'm not scared...'
>
> (Deborah)

Although the legal issues and procedures are clear, George and Hutton point out how hard it is for a parent to tolerate or agree to their son's or daughter's refusal of treatment, and that the implementation of the decision-making process may have to accommodate 'oscillation in psychological/emotional capacity' (2003: 2664). They say that the resulting exacerbation of both disputes and symptoms may spill over into the ward and become distressing for staff and other patients as well as the young person and the parents. However, this complex set of dynamics may be managed more readily in the specialist environment where expertise at handling such a difficult situation is likely to be greater. According to George and Hutton, despite the horror and distress of a young person's cancer journey and as unwelcome as their impending death may be, if the process is managed properly through skilled specialist input, the experience can be 'meaningful, productive and even "healthy"' (2003: 2663).

The preservation of fertility

While it may eventually be necessary to negotiate end-of-life decision-making, at the outset of the illness the hope must be of long-term survival, thus the threat to future fertility is a matter of some urgency and the issue of fertility preservation must be addressed. Yet Guy Makin's (University of Manchester 2006) study of young male cancer patients indicates that while boys as young as 13 are capable of producing semen samples with normal sperm counts, a study of childless male cancer survivors found that although 77 per cent of them from 14–40 would like to be able to father children in the future, only half had been given the option of banking sperm. This accords with the evidence presented in the last chapter on the lack of reliability of offering sperm banking routinely to all eligible males (Reebals et al. 2006). Thus, according to Dr Makin, it is important to train medical professionals to discuss the issue (University of Manchester 2006) as if sperm collection became routine, later regrets about infertility might be avoided.

However, Wallace and Brougham (2005: 141) claim that semen cryopreservation is particularly problematic in adolescence; there are few adolescent-friendly facilities and sperm banking is not universally practised in paediatric oncology centres. Thus what may be experienced as embarrassing needs to be routinized so that the option is offered as a matter of course rather than the adolescent or their family having to seek it out.

The issue is complex for young women; the procedures for egg harvesting may not be readily understood or available at local levels. Nevertheless, the routine shielding of the ovaries during radiotherapy and the collection and cryopreservation of mature oocytes will at least give some hope for future procreation. The complexity of the challenges posed by the threat to fertility was discussed in detail in the last chapter. Suffice it to say here that hope for future fertility preservation may give both young men and women an additional incentive to fight the illness. At the very least it may encourage compliance with treatment that might otherwise be refused if no hope for procreation can be offered.

Supporting staff

While the focus of this volume has been on the experiences of the young adults with cancer, there are inevitably issues relating to the support and training of professionals in such a potentially demanding situation. Staff on the specialist ward are described by Geehan as: 'emotional "rocks" who understood whatever we were feeling and were always strong when ever things got a little too much for us and would never break down in front of us' (2003: 2681). However, such support does not come without personal cost and staff need both training and support to be able to sustain the continuous and continuing demands on their sensibilities.

Bearison's (2006) study shows that a survey of paediatric oncologists in the USA found a serious lack of training in end-of-life care and that this same lack of attention was manifested in a range of medical text books that had 'little helpful information' (Bearison 2006: 214). Nevertheless Bearison acknowledges that while such training should be integral to professional education, no amount of classroom discussion, role play, reading or discussion can truly prepare for the experience he describes as 'emotionally draining and heart wrenching' (2006: 25).

While the hope must be of cure, not all the young people will survive their cancers, yet medical staff are trained to 'expect to save each and every child'. The death of a young person appears so unnatural in modern Western society that the impact can be far-reaching. Professionals not only have to deal with their sense of failure and loss, they are also required to provide compassion to the family and to move on to the care of the next child. According to Bearison, there is no standard or canonical procedure to best support staff, some need to talk, others need distraction, some might prefer professional support within the care setting, while others favour extra-mural activities that help them bond with colleagues (2006: 184). Bearison argues that counselling should not be imposed upon staff and that institutional interventions are unwarranted. However, the opportunities to speak with colleagues and the chance to meet outside the hospital setting to 'reinvigorate their collegiality and to develop and maintain interpersonal relations in roles other than strictly hospital care is an appealing idea' (Bearison 2006: 263). How practical this is in reality may be questionable given shift work, family commitments and the many factors that limit the ease of socializing outside the workplace, thus it may be that support structures need to be in place primarily within the care setting. Morgan and Hubber recognize the demands placed on staff supporting young people on a specialist unit:

> Experiencing the relapse and death of teenagers can cause staff to become very demoralized. It is very important, therefore, to have a

support network for all professionals working with these patients, because only then are they able to support the other patients who are also struggling with this aspect.

(2004: 134)

I was told by Simon, the learning mentor on the specialist ward, of the valuable help given during supervision sessions during which the emotional demands of the job could be addressed and shared and support offered, particularly after traumatic events. In addition, regular support meetings allow staff to interact less formally than in 'case meetings', and offer as Simon said, 'just a chance for people to vent their feelings'.

Outside the specialist setting, staff tend to find young adults 'demanding' in a number of ways, at least in part because of the life stage issues addressed throughout this volume. Indeed, in Bearison's (2006) research on the demands of palliative care for dying children of all ages from infancy upwards, the instances recalled by staff are disproportionately represented by cancers in teenagers, suggesting that these cases might have presented particularly traumatic and difficult challenges. Thus if models of good practice are to be implemented successfully outside the specialist setting, it is not only the philosophy of care for the young adults that needs to be embedded into practice; the support of staff must become part of the culture.

The importance of non-medical professionals

The centrality of the role of medical professionals and others involved directly in health care is obvious, but the significance of non-medical professionals became clear to me both through my observations on the ward and via the interview data collected from the young people. Simon, the learning mentor on the TCT ward, holds a relatively recent appointment made in recognition of the special needs of young people. He acknowledged that the age range is wide – from 13 to 25 – and this represents a correspondingly wide range of needs. Despite this, he identified unifying characteristics, for example, even if the patient had left full-time education and did not need assistance with home tutoring, there was still the prospect of career change and planning for the future to be addressed:

> We try and make sure as much as we can that people can carry on with their education while they're going through their treatment ... and for the ones who aren't in education sometimes [we] can re-evaluate what they're doing and [if they] want to get into education. So I can help them apply for college courses or university courses; give them some career advice and help with the application proce-

dure ... and that's really good for giving them something to focus on. It's something that's a link back into normal life, and something that's going to happen at the end of their treatment.

(Simon)

While they are on the ward, all the young people can benefit from the input and support of a learning mentor, but once they have left the relative security of the specialist care environment they may find themselves in a potentially hostile and challenging situation. We have already seen through the testimonies of the young people that looking different or losing touch with a peer group can lead to distressing social situations and Simon suggested that those in this age group are probably the ones that find it most difficult to re-integrate:

You get stories of teachers whipping people's baseball caps off the heads, saying, 'You're not allowed to wear hats in schools' and then you're really fighting a losing battle to build up their confidence again from that, because that's such a damaging, damaging thing. I heard that one girl on her first day at high school had that happen to her, on her first day at this new school ... a group of liaison nurses visit schools to try and make the school aware of all the different issues around the patient so that hopefully things like that don't happen.

(Simon)

This example is redolent of Ricky's experience recounted in Chapter 5 that resulted in his return to school lasting for only two days and suggests that liaison work is essential to ensure that teaching staff are aware of the issues and handle the young people's insecurities with sensitivity. Liaison work may also be extended to the peer group in school; visits to the hospital could be encouraged to prevent the difficulties in re-establishing friendships at a later stage which presents a risk if contact has been lost. As Craig (2006) says, if young adults have been isolated from their peer group, and have become dependent on parents for companionship, as well as physical support, this can result in their subsequent unwillingness to take part in activities away from the security of the family. They can be afraid of failure and believe 'it may be better not to try than to prove it is impossible' (Craig 2006: 110), thus everything should be done to maximize the chance of reintegration. Re-assurance that the patients' friends will be welcome on the ward and some preparation about what they might expect when they visit can help to maintain the links so vital to later social and emotional recovery.

We have seen that the learning mentor in the specialist care environment has a key role in offering non-clinical support. Yet there are other professional groups who contribute to the care and support of the young adult with cancer who can offer many benefits. Through a discussion with Cat, one of only a few Activity Co-ordinators in the UK, the key importance of that role became clear. Cat talked of the need for the young patients to undertake as many 'normal' activities as possible, thus maintaining links with youth culture and boosting morale. Her remit was to organize events within the ward such as music workshops, chill out sessions (yoga, etc.), a website project, film nights with take-aways, games and coffee mornings; and community-based activities outside the hospital such as dance projects, golf and a pool tournament. A music project spanned both the ward and the community, providing studio, sound and film courses, recording sessions and the opportunity to learn a musical instrument. While such activities may be dismissed as simply 'keeping the young people occupied', it is likely that offering such opportunities has a far more profound effect on outcomes if the chance of compliance is increased through accommodating the social and emotional needs of the young people. The key importance of this role is reflected on by Geehan whose own experience demonstrates its significance in contributing to the deeply symbolic sense of 'normality' that has been a concept raised many times by the young people throughout this volume:

> One of the most influential people in our Unit is the activities co-ordinator. Her role is immensely important, as she is not only there to try and get us all out of bed in the morning, but in trying to get a group of teenagers who are feeling less than fantastic, motivated and excited about an activity . . . she boosts morale and helps to maintain some semblance of normality.
>
> (Geehan 2003: 2682)

The value of the roles held by Cat and Simon seems clear; however, the relevance of some support staff may not be understood and can even be challenged by medical personnel outside the specialist setting. Without adequate recognition of the social needs of cancer patients and their families and an integrated multi disciplinary approach to care, non-medical professionals working with the young adults and their families may find their role marginalized by medical professionals who see only the illness and the imperative of medical intervention. Indeed, it seems that in some non-specialist centres medical staff do not understand why a social worker may be helpful as the profession may be associated with 'problem families'. An interview conducted with Hazel, a medical social worker at a disease-specific centre, indicated that she sometimes experienced difficulties in convincing medical staff that her role was of any relevance. Yet several hundred miles from where Hazel works, by chance, a mother who was present during my interview with her son, referred to Hazel as having been pivotal in the family's ability to access support and services once they returned to their home. A specialist social worker may be able to access sources of support and funding of which professionals in a non-specialist care environment are unaware.

However, discussions with parents resulted in them admitting that at first they had felt stigmatized by being allocated a 'social worker', and despite their appreciation of their social worker's contribution, they wished he or she had been called a 'key worker' or 'support co-ordinator' as this would have made the family seem less of a 'problem' family. Indeed, the centrality of a key worker is a major recommendation in the NICE Guidance (2005a).

Extending good practice across other care settings

Morgan and Hubber (2004) ask whether it is the location or the philosophy of care that matters. While the best practice has been found in the specialist care setting, there have nevertheless been examples of good practice outside this environment, thus indicating its potential to exist beyond the specialist unit. Realistically, the funding for all patients in the age range to be treated in specialist care settings is unlikely to be forthcoming in the near future, thus having identified the essence of success in the specialist setting, ways need to be found to extend it into the non-specialist environment. As Morgan and Hubber (2004: 138) conclude, 'this philosophy of caring can be applied to other units by a motivated team of professionals'. If age-appropriate care can be rolled out across the health service through training and outreach work, or if doctors can undertake an element of their training in the specialist setting, the philosophy can be taken out into wider healthcare provision.

According to Thomas (2006), healthcare professionals outside the specialist setting report greater difficulty in talking to young people than they do any other age group and Thomas claims there is evidence that health professionals avoid the discussion of emotionally charged issues with young adults. From the evidence presented in this volume, we can see that in the specialist care setting staff have developed an expertise in relating to the young people not just at the superficial level of banter and joking, but they are also able to engage at a deeper level and discuss the very real fears and concerns held by the young people about their illnesses, treatments and futures. As discussed in Chapter 3, the jokey and informal atmosphere is carefully managed in order to ensure that professional boundaries are maintained, and, as Arbuckle et al. (2005) acknowledge, the training of staff in this expertise is essential.

Thomas reflects on how best practice might be extended in the Australian context. He suggests that:

One of the ways we could address this issue is to provide specialized medical and psychological support remotely, by encouraging local clinicians to work with others with expertise in the area ... one model is that the patient's case would be reviewed by local clinicians in conjunction with a group embodying wider expertise, resulting in a comprehensive management plan. This approach would result in standardized treatment based on best practice and would be expected to enhance health outcomes. Online support using Web-based resources, may also be a powerful way of ensuring that both local clinical treatment and psychosocial supports remain on track.

(2006: 1)

Morgan and Hubber (2004) suggest that 'virtual units' should be developed. However, the way in which they use the term 'virtual' does not signify a web-based or electronic network, rather, it refers to a peripatetic group of expert professionals filling the gap in non-specialist settings by taking the philosophy of the specialist ward into the wider healthcare environment. Yet Simon (learning mentor) acknowledged that when undertaking outreach work it was not unusual to meet with resistance from professionals who were being asked to consider delivering care differently. Thus to what extent the input of the virtual unit changes the culture in the non-specialist setting is not yet clear. As Morgan and Hubber acknowledge, this strategy is likely to challenge existing practice and as a result is almost certain to be contentious. Merely providing expert advice and support through a specialist network, outreach work or on the Web can only make an impact if local practitioners accept the basic principle that young people do indeed have very particular characteristics and needs and that practice may need to change to accommodate them.

One professional situated outside the specialist setting who had clearly accepted that young adults have specific needs was Alison, the lead cancer nurse in a general hospital. She recognized in her (relatively few) young adult patients many of the issues of isolation and 'difference' addressed throughout this book and discussed 'shared care' as an approach to their treatment:

The majority of young people that I've cared for have experienced shared care. Where maybe they've undergone diagnostic procedure in the district general hospital, then had a specialist intervention at a unit somewhere else in the country where the treatment plan has been recommended and then they've come back and had the treatment delivered locally ... the young people must be made aware that they are not alone and that there are other [young] people and potentially be put in contact. Which is why I think that sometimes the shared care is beneficial, where they will spend time [in] out-patient clinics and see that they are not alone. There is close liaison with the consultant staff ... and quite often when there [are] clinical specialists involved in the disease group, then the clinical nurse specialist at the specialist centre and a specialist at the district general hospital will liaise with each other. And that information will then be transmitted from the nurse specialist to the oncology unit, and also to the district nurses and to the GP and other health professionals involved also including the family and the extended family.

(Alison)

We can see how this model may address some of the clinical issues, and it may even be that the approach can extend inclusion in clinical trials to general hospitals. However, Alison acknowledged that in the shared care model, the delivery of treatment locally would separate the young people from their peers, as she said: 'The risk of that is they're getting the same treatment as they would do in a specialist unit, but they're more isolated from their peer group.' This indicates that even if the philosophy of the age-specific unit can be implemented in the non-specialist setting, the young people will remain isolated from their peers. The value of peer support is clear from the testimonies of the young adults and in Geehan's reflections on her stay in a TCT unit: 'When fighting cancer at a young age, it is immensely valuable to be surrounded by others of a similar age' (2003: 2682). Nevertheless, until age-appropriate care is available to all, the shared care option would still appear to offer at least some contact with peers and is likely to be a considerable improvement on the negative experiences recounted by some participants.

Conclusion

The aim of the research was to reach a largely unstudied group of people, many of whose needs have remained unmet (Albritton and Bleyer 2003). Through entering the life world of the young adult with cancer, I have attempted to capture the essence of what it is like to be a young adult with cancer and to glimpse the meaning of the experience for the participants, thus identifying how provision to support them through the cancer journey can best be delivered.

What the preceding testimonies have established is that the age group has specific needs and the accounts have identified what these consist of in the young people's own terms rather than relying on an interpretation from parents or professionals. Some of the topics covered in the book relate directly to issues raised in the NICE Guidance (2005a) and can thus help to inform policy, others are more personally orientated, but nevertheless still contribute to a necessary understanding of what the young person is facing and what might affect their compliance and thus the eventual outcome.

It is clear that there is much good practice, particularly in the specialist centres, and that staff in these centres of excellence have a sound grasp of the issues and a deep understanding of the experiences that the young people are going through, yet as we have seen, 'evidence' of this has hitherto been regarded as 'anecdotal'. What this volume offers is evidence based on personal accounts organized in a way that is designed to act as an accessible reference point for those who are charged with the care of young adults in whatever setting. I also hope it provides a contribution to the 'proof' required by those who are responsible for the design and implementation of policy.

It seems likely that the testimonies in this volume will come as no surprise to staff in the specialist care setting, yet, according to Morgan and Hubber (2004), medical opinion about adolescent units still varies enormously and many doctors are reluctant to refer their patients to such a unit. Similarly, Lewis (2005: 241) suggests that the concept of specialist units still generates controversy and that 'some clinicians doubt the need to consider teenagers and young adults as an identifiable and separate group' and believe that 'the group should be managed within the context of site-specific teams'. It is to be hoped that the first-hand accounts included in this volume will speak clearly to the reader of the significance of life stage and of the particular need that it carries with it when travelling the cancer journey, and, as a consequence, the central importance of incorporating age-specific awareness and expertise into the care setting, be it specialist or non-specialist, will be accepted. The case for age-appropriate care seems compelling, but are patient numbers sufficient to justify such provision? According to Michelagnoli et al. (2003: 2571), the epidemiological data are 'persuasive of a "critical mass", not just reflecting patient numbers but highlighting a huge "unmet" need'.

Finally, much of this volume has focused on the treatment period, but, as Neville (2000) points out, the journey does not end when treatment ceases, and the ramifications may be felt for years. However, Decker et al. (2004: 332) report 'survivors' lack of knowledge about late effects and lack of awareness of their risks'. While Viner (2003) is aware of the danger of 'over-medicalising' well survivors, he argues that they may nevertheless benefit from long-term support to deal with physical and psychosocial late effects; hence ongoing opportunities to talk through the experience should be made available. Thomas et al. (2006) say lower levels of family cohesion are experienced by adolescent cancer survivors; this is therefore a group that need to have a safety net in place for a possibly lengthy period after recovery in order that their physical healing can be matched by social and psychological healing.

Key points

- Despite their differences, young adults have particular age-related needs.

- There is more that unites young adults than divides them.

- Young adults do not fit easily within adult or children's care settings.

- Staff in non-specialist settings can find young adults challenging.

- The philosophy of care in the specialist setting can improve compliance.

- Issues of concern to young adults are understood in the specialist setting.

- Inclusion in clinical trials – more likely in the specialist setting – may improve outcomes.

- Managing the family's role and consent procedures may be more familiar in the specialist setting.

- Fertility issues may be more skilfully handled in the specialist setting.

- Staff caring for young adults with cancer need both training and support.

- Support staff in the specialist centres are recognized as key members of the team.

- Good practice can be rolled out across non-specialist settings.

- Virtual units, peripatetic teams and shared care can be adopted to good effect.

Notes

1   I have not gathered data that can show that non-compliance is higher among those not treated in a specialist setting; indeed (apart from Emma) all those I interviewed in this category were by definition in treatment or follow-up in the non-specialist setting as they were recruited by professionals involved in their care. Yet, as a result of this, they may be unrepresentative of the wider population.

2   The centrality of the contribution of non-medical professionals who contribute to the multi disciplinary team is discussed later in this chapter.

Appendix I Methods

At the outset of the present research project in 2005, I assumed that I could replicate the method used to gather data from the parents of young adults with cancer. This had consisted of distributing an appeal via health professionals and through the cancer networks in newsletters and other publications. This method had proved highly satisfactory in terms of the responses from a range of parents. Not only were the resulting qualitative data rich and detailed, the approach also allowed parents to choose how and when to contribute. It situated the power with them, they could write as and when they felt able, pick up and put down their narrative account as it suited them without any pressure from a researcher arriving for a pre-arranged interview at a time they might have felt unequal to the task. Thus it appeared to be not only a productive, but also an ethical way in which to collect data of such a sensitive nature with the high risk of causing distress to participants (Grinyer and Thomas 2001; Grinyer 2002a; 2004a; 2004b). In the light of all these points it seemed appropriate to continue with a similar approach directed at young adults themselves as approved by my university department's ethics committee.

The initial attempt to reach the young adults was through a weekend organized by the Teenage Cancer Trust for past and current young adults with cancer. The organizers were hopeful that the inclusion of a flyer in all the delegate packs, coupled with a few strategically placed large posters, would result in a significant number of replies. However, despite the best efforts of all concerned, I received only three contributions as detailed in Box A.1.

So, if the young people were not going to come to me – or at least send their narratives – then I would have to go to them. The sole option for reaching such a cohort was through their treatment centres, and this would involve going through the MREC (Multi-site Research Ethics Committee) process, a lengthy and time-consuming procedure but one that appeared to be essential if the research was to succeed.

Clearly ethical issues are enormously important in all research, but in this area they are particularly pertinent where the scope for causing harm or distress is manifold. It is only in recent years that the ethical practices embedded into research have come under scrutiny and have been subject to processes designed to 'measure' their ethics. Much has been written about the LRECs (Local Research Ethics Committee) and MRECs through which all research proposals to gather data in a healthcare setting are scrutinized. Questions have been asked as to the 'real' purpose of the committees: are they

Box A.1 Details of participants

Narratives were submitted by:

Devika: At school when diagnosed with acute lymphoblastic leukaemia.

Gemma: A nurse on an orthopaedic ward, 23 when diagnosed with lymphoma (also interviewed).

James: At school when diagnosed with acute lymphoblastic leukaemia at 16.

Narratives not contributed as a response to the appeal:

Ruth: At school when diagnosed at 14 with anaplastic large cell lymphoma, Ruth submitted a previously written account.

Steve: A student in his early twenties, a long-term survivor of childhood cancer diagnosed when he was 10.

(The narratives from Ruth and Steve were sent as a result of pre-existing personal contact.)

---

really for the protection of participants or are they attempts to stifle research and prevent litigation? Even if they are not intended to stifle research, this has in many cases been the result as the time-consuming nature of the process and its attendant bureaucracy act an inhibitor to all but the most determined and those with the institutional support and a time scale sufficient to see the procedure through. As Richard Smith said in an editorial in the *BMJ*:

> Do you need approval from an ethics committee to ring up chief executives of hospitals and ask them questions? As a journalist, a member of parliament, or a confidence trickster you wouldn't, but if you are a researcher who has drawn up a protocol you might. Ethics committees, which were devised to protect vulnerable patients from some abuse, have forgotten why they were created and have begun to equate chief executives with the unconscious or the mentally incompetent. They have in other words spun out of control.
>
> (2004: 7460)

Smith continues by talking about the 'frustration, anger and even despair' among researchers required to undergo such processes. Writing on what he calls the 'bizarre obstacles' put in the way of researchers Brindle (2005) evokes Euripides and says that those whom the gods wish to destroy they first make mad, and that it is tempting to conclude that this is the strategy employed by the deities at the Department of Health who wish to destroy health services research. Brindle cites examples of academics who have had to undergo repeated police checks and even blood tests for studies that involve no contact with patients. He also refers to one case where the paperwork for the Multi-site Ethics Committee procedure ran to 6,000 pages, weighed 34kg, took a researcher eight months full-time work to negotiate but still had to be cleared by the research governance process at local level in 62 separate locations.

However, Research Ethics Committees, while tedious and time-consuming, do offer legitimacy. As Hallowell et al. (2005) say, having been through such a process lends a certain credibility to our research and may make access easier to negotiate simply because, for example in the health field, any hospital Trust approached with the MREC approval knows that we must be serious and credible researchers. Yet, as Hallowell et al. also point out:

> We believe that this bureaucratization of research ethics raises a . . . serious problem. We suggest that as 'ethical approval' emerges as the supposed benchmark test for 'guaranteeing' that our research projects are ethical, research ethics is in danger of becoming removed from actual research practice. Research ethics is increasingly seen as an 'add-on', a rubber-stamping exercise that we must undergo (with gritted teeth), rather than as an integral and ongoing aspect of our research.
>
> (2005: 144)

Indeed, the ethics of undertaking research on such a topic and with this age group does present some challenging ethical problems. 'Harm' is acknowledged by Alderson and Morrow (2004: 35) often to be 'invisible and elusive'. As they say, while medical research can seriously harm people, in contrast, social researchers believe their work to be largely benign (2004: 36), yet intrusion into the lives of their participants still has the potential for causing harm and distress. I would add that in the health field this effect can be exacerbated. The ethics of conducting research in such a sensitive area with young people who may be vulnerable both physically and emotionally was a constant concern. There are many ethical issues relating to research with young people that are more problematic than with adults. Among concerns identified are those that relate to obtaining informed consent and the preparation of age-specific information sheets; the need to protect participants from harm as adults' definitions of harm may vary from those of young people, and some harms may only be known in the longer term. The participants must feel confident enough to refuse or withdraw from the research and know how to contact the researcher to make enquiries or complain. Mindful of these concerns, certain safeguards were built into the research design in order to minimize the chance that any young person would be harmed by the experience.

The inclusion and exclusion criteria as approved by the ethics committee were clear, and in both Trusts prospective participants were identified by staff as suitable both physically and emotionally for inclusion according to these criteria. Participants were given an approved information sheet before they agreed to an interview. This informed them of their rights to withdraw at any stage and emphasized that withdrawal would in no way be questioned or affect their future treatment. Details of how and why the data would be used were provided and it was made clear who would have access to the interview material. Should they become distressed or concerned, provision was made for support staff to speak to them if they wished. In the event, no participant expressed any concern or anxiety either before, during or after the interview, all had my contact details should they wish to withdraw their accounts or ask further questions. No participant did this. However, some asked for further details of how the interview data would be used.

In the field

In the specialist care setting

Once approvals had been given, the reality of the challenge had to be faced. I had known that this would be a hard-to-reach group, but had been un-prepared for how slowly the data would be gathered. My plans to visit the TCT ward had to be changed on several occasions, I could not go if I had a cold or sore throat in case of passing on infection to the patients who had lowered immunity, and cancellation of some visits occurred for this reason. On other occasions, I had arranged to go to the ward only to have a phone call a day or two earlier to say that none of the patients would be well enough to talk to me. On another visit I arrived at the ward to find that all the patients who had agreed to participate were asleep, I was asked to come back three hours later and though by the time I returned they had awoken, two were too ill to see me and the third fell asleep while I was talking to her, I left the ward with only one complete interview, though on that occasion I also talked informally to a mother and the sister of one young woman too ill to participate.

After a visit to the TCT ward that resulted in a single successful interview it was suggested to me by one of the doctors on the ward that I contact outpatients' clinics where I would have access to young people who had completed their treatment who would not be so ill. However, all the clinic consultants felt that the patients were already participating in enough re-search (though what type of research was not specified) and I was denied access.

The interviews in the specialist hospital ward took place in the day room or the 'quiet room' away from the bustle of the ward or in the participant's room if they were too ill to leave their bed. If a parent – usually the mother – was present, she too would be invited to attend the interview and contribute, thus conforming to Arksey's (1996) definition of a joint interview with all its concomitant effects on rapport, the contribution of different kinds of knowledge and filling in each other's gaps. Nevertheless, the presence of a parent may also have had a constraining effect in some instances. I also spoke to members of the ward staff both formally and informally, thus gaining the perspective of those caring for the young adults. All participants were asked if they would like their own names used if quoted in publication or if they would like to select a pseudonym: only one participant chose an alternative name.

Research on the ward was predominantly based on interview data. However being 'on the ward' for several days at a time meant that while not undertaking an ethnographic study in the traditional sense of the term, I was able to make a number of observations about the environment and absorb the atmosphere. In a rare moment of true participant observation in which I was able to participate in the ward activities, (observer as participant, Robson 1995), I took part in a music therapy 'jam session' with a visiting musician, ward staff, a parent and patients on the ward. This allowed me more informal contact with patients and staff and contributed to my ability to immerse myself in the field.

Box A.2 offers some details of the participants on the TCT ward.

In the non-specialist care setting

The interviews in the non-specialist Trust were sporadic and unpredictable in their frequency as I was able only to respond to local staff informing me that a patient, identified by them and in the age group, had agreed to participate. Despite the fact that qualitative methods do not require large numbers of participants, the slowness of the data collection and the unpredictability of recruitment were at times dispiriting, but while patients recruited from the non-specialist Trust were few and far between, staff were immensely helpful in identifying those who fulfilled the inclusion criteria and in putting me in touch with them.

The interviews with those young people not treated in a specialist centre took place in a variety of locations as all the participants were either in re-covery or being treated as outpatients. Those in the participant's home led to other family members being drawn into the discussion thus providing the additional perspective of a joint interview (Arksey 1996). As in the specialist environment, although the presence of others may have led to the young person being guarded in what they said, this did not appear to be the case.

Though recruited from a Trust with no specialist facilities, this did not mean that the participant had not been treated on a TCT ward or equivalent

Box A.2 Participants from the TCT ward

Aidan (and his mother): At school when diagnosed at 15 with osteosarcoma in his pelvis.

Dawn: A hairdresser diagnosed at 20 with acute lymphoblastic leukaemia.

Donovan: At college doing a joinery course when diagnosed with osteosarcoma at 17.

Hoody (and his parents): At school when diagnosed with osteosarcoma at the age of 16.

Lucy (and her mother): At school when diagnosed at 13 with lymphoma.

Luke (and his aunt): At school when diagnosed at 16 with Ewing's sarcoma in his hip.

Nathan: Apprentice joiner and at college when diagnosed at 17 with Hodgkin's disease.

Ricky (and his mother): At school when diagnosed with leukaemia at the age of 15.

Ross (and his partner Hannah): A self-employed agricultural/haulage contractor when diagnosed with osteosarcoma at 23.

Thomas: At school when diagnosed with osteosarcoma in his knee.

Toni (and her mother): About to go to university when diagnosed at 19 with lymphoma.

Vicky (and her mother): At school when diagnosed at 15 with leukaemia.

---

as some had been sent outside the Trust area for treatment to a specialist care setting. Thus accounts from this group are based on a wider range of experience of settings of care than I had initially anticipated. Similarly, some of the participants from the specialist ward had also been treated in a non-specialist care setting, thus they were able to offer a degree of comparison between the different environments

Box A.3 offers some details of the participants from outside the specialist ward.

Box A.3 Participants from the non-specialist Trust

Adrian (and his partner Cindy's mother): A scaffolder diagnosed at 18 with testicular cancer, living with his girlfriend Cindy and her parents.

Charlotte (and her grandmother): At college when diagnosed at 17 with a liver tumour.

Craig: Diagnosed at 18 with testicular cancer.

Emma (and her partner Gary and children Brooklyn and Chloe): A full-time mother when diagnosed at 21 with Hodgkin's lymphoma.

Gemma: A nurse on an orthopaedic ward when diagnosed at 23 with Hodgkin's lymphoma.

Kelly (and her infant daughter): A wife and mother of a baby when diagnosed at 26 with lymphoma.

Marc: An apprentice in a factory and at college doing an HND when diagnosed at 20 with testicular cancer.

Mark: A butcher already married when diagnosed with testicular cancer at 21.

Michelle (and her mother): Newly graduated from university when diagnosed with an adrenal tumour at 21.

Nicola: A play worker with infants and pregnant when diagnosed at 19 with an ovarian tumour.

Philip: A trainee Outward Bound instructor when diagnosed at 20 with bowel cancer.

Steven: A heavy goods vehicle apprentice when diagnosed at 18 with Hodgkin's disease.

Though an element of participant observation was possible, interviewing provided the overwhelming majority of data. The symbolic interactionist approach to interviewing regards the interview as a social event based on mutual participant observation in which there is no clear distinction between research interviews and other forms of social interaction (Fielding 1995). Thus the interviews were conducted as informally and conversationally as possible, though as Grbich (1999: 86) warns:

> The notion of a friendly conversation implies an established relationship with some form of reciprocity. Although this may well be achievable in some situations, in others it is an overglorification of the power-laden, awkward interchanges that actually occur.

While I took heed of Grbich's concerns and in most instances I believe I succeeded in establishing a rapport with the participants by using an unstructured approach that allowed participants to identify areas of importance to them, a very small minority offered limited responses to my questions. Nevertheless, the majority of the interviews generated rich and detailed accounts of the experience that allow a glimpse of the lived reality.

Atkin et al. (2006) suggest that work in the field of young people and illness experiences rarely addresses ethnic minority families, and I must acknowledge that this applies to my research. Only one young woman, Sunita, was from an Asian family, but it was her sister to whom I talked as Sunita was too ill to participate. While this omission is regrettable, the demographics and ethnic identities of the young people both willing and able to participate dictated the characteristics of the sample. Indeed, no participant was selected by me, of those in the medical setting all were recruited by staff in whose care they were, but further work among ethnic minorities should be encouraged in future research.

I understood that I would be interviewing young people at various stages of their cancer journey; some would be very ill and unlikely to recover while others would be uncertain what their future held. Though I prepared myself as well as I could for this difficult task, in the event the interviewing process was a profoundly moving experience. Each interview had a different dynamic; to a large extent I let the participants dictate the nature and content of the interview. Using a grounded theory approach (Glaser and Strauss 1967), I also took back into the field topics and questions that had been raised in interviews with previous participants. The interviews led to some emotional encounters during which I was entrusted with the deepest fears of the participant, as well as being told funny stories and accounts of struggles with officialdom that made me angry on their behalf. To remain emotionally disengaged was impossible and thus presented a challenge in terms of limiting subjectivity and bias. While objectivity may never be attainable, it seems that under these circumstances it becomes even more elusive. Nevertheless, while through a process of reflexivity I acknowledge my positionality I have, through the analysis, tried to give voice to the young people in an attempt to convey the experience.

In addition to the interviews with the young adults, key health professionals were interviewed. As well as the formal interviews, many informal discussions with staff took place and the information collected through this method forms a context that acts as wider basis for some of the comments and observations made throughout the text. Those interviewed formally are shown in Box A.4.

Box A.4 Professionals interviewed formally

> **Alison**: Lead cancer nurse in a non-specialist setting.
>
> **Cat**: Activity coordinator on the specialist ward.
>
> **Deborah**: Staff nurse on the specialist ward.
>
> **Diane**: Sister on the specialist ward.
>
> **Hazel**: Medical social worker in a non-specialist setting.
>
> **Dr James**: General practitioner at a university practice.
>
> **Simon**: Learning mentor on the specialist ward.
>
> **Sue**: Lead Macmillan clinical nurse specialist for teenagers and young adults.

Although I have used the term 'interview' to describe the method, it might be described as incorporating a 'narrative' approach. Bearison (2006: 20) argues that 'eliciting narratives is very different from conducting interviews'. The distinction drawn by Bearison suggests that within an interview the interviewer's questions inevitably shape the answer, but in contrast the narrative approach shifts the balance to participant who selects the topic, issues and focus. While the researcher may probe by asking 'tell me more about that' and asking for clarification, the approach remains essentially non-directive. It was my intention to situate the power and control with the young people in the 'interview' situation, and encourage them to focus on what had been of significance to them, but by taking issues back into the field I was in some instances additionally guiding the process at points during the interaction. Thus it seems that a purist narrative approach would have been difficult to achieve, and the data as a result were produced from a combination of interviewing and narrative approaches.

Analysis

Data were collected until saturation had been reached. Glaser and Strauss (1967) refer to this process as 'theoretical saturation', this refers to the point at which observations no longer serve to question or modify theories generated from earlier data (May 1997: 144). In order to make such a judgement, the collection of qualitative data incorporates a process of ongoing analysis throughout the data collection period (Robson 1995). When new issues are raised by a participant, these can be taken out into subsequent interviews, thus while the topics have been generated by the interviewees in the first instance, the researcher can use them as the basis for a topic guide for future interviews.

While the researcher is constantly developing an analytical framework throughout the process, it is nevertheless crucial that analytical transparency and rigour are demonstrated if qualitative data are to avoid being dismissed as 'merely anecdotal' or highly selective. Mindful of such a requirement, the data were rigorously analysed using methods of data reduction, display and conclusion drawing (Miles and Huberman 1994). Miles and Huberman note that extended text is dispersed, poorly structured and extremely bulky, and that in order to avoid jumping to unfounded conclusions, or over-weighting a particularly dramatic passage, certain processes must be observed during analysis. To this end the data have been subjected to codification. They have been sorted and sifted in a manner that facilitates the identification of similar phrases, themes and patterns. Through the identification of commonalties and differences, and a consideration of the relationship between the variables, a set of generalizations was gradually developed to cover the consistencies discerned in the database.

The chapter headings reflect these themes and though they are overlapping and interconnected, arising as they do from material that is unstructured, there has been an attempt to organize them into a coherent structure that allows a degree of analysis and ease of access to the reader. Though the original words of participants can be so powerful that it can be tempting to allow them to speak for themselves, and there are thus many original words cited, the quotes were selected from a substantial data set and in most cases typify responses.

Appendix II Extract from A. Grinyer (2002a) *Cancer in Young Adults: Through Parents' Eyes*

The term adopted by Apter (2001) for those aged 18–24 years is 'thresholders'. This is a highly descriptive and relevant way in which to interpret this life-stage. Apter argues that there are expectations from the young people themselves, their parents, teachers and employers that after the age of 18 they will be mature and self-sufficient. The result of this expectation and consequent separation from family is that 'thresholders' become reliant to a much greater extent on friends, yet these friends do not have the stability to act as a substitute for family support. As they too are in transitional phases they tend to let each other down, argue with each other and move away in search of employment. Yet many of these young people will encounter major problems – not necessarily health related – and because of the weakening of their family bonds may be reluctant to turn to their parents for assistance.

Apter argues that parenting a teenager is not the same as parenting a thresholder. Not only are they caught half-way between dependence and independence, they seem mature enough to have their problems under control, but in reality they are rarely mature enough to actually solve them. Despite this immaturity, Apter suggests that thresholders want to protect parents and appreciate the financial difficulties they might have.

The age group addressed in research undertaken by Brannen, Dodd, Oakley and Storey (1994) is limited to 15–17 year olds, however, even at this younger end of the age range, they suggest that young people are moving towards greater social and economic independence. Despite the suggestion by Apter (2001) that the parenting of a teenager is qualitatively different, according to Brannen and colleagues's research findings (1994) it appears that many of the same 'threshold' issues arise. This is evidenced by their findings that a quarter of their respondents considered themselves to be 'adult', half claimed to be 'in between' and a quarter did not think of themselves as 'adult'. Thus we can see that the transitional nature of this life-stage in which childhood has not yet been fully left behind, but neither has adulthood been fully realized, is arguably characterized by a struggle for independence. This concept is of central importance as the impact of serious illness may have a profound effect on the young person's attempt at establishing independence.

The psychological models of adolescent development drawn upon by

Brannen and colleagues suggest that adolescence is also a time of emotional turbulence. It will come as no surprise to anyone who has lived through their children's teenage years that the parents in this study used terms such as 'moody', 'depressed' and 'ratty' to describe the behaviour of their adolescent children. In addition, these authors suggest that adolescence is a life-stage when young people are expected to exhibit rudeness and rebelliousness, have no respect for their parents and refuse to listen to adult advice (1994: 27). According to Brannen and colleagues teenagers are emotional because they are at a stage where they are renegotiating relationships with their parents, and making new peer group and sexual relationships. This can weaken family bonds as young people seek the company of their peers away from parental supervision, again a manifestation of the search for independence (1994: 131).

During this period of young adulthood when independence is being sought, relationships with parents in all aspects of family life are being renegotiated. Thus even when a young adult is well, parents' attempts to regulate behaviour can have implications for young people's health and health-related behaviour (Brannen, Dodd, Oakley and Storey 1994: 126). However, when a young adult is diagnosed with an illness, the relationship with parents can be thrown into crisis. The type of illnesses referred to by these authors tend to be sore throats, colds and 'flu. If such minor illnesses as these can impact upon family dynamics, how much greater must the impact be when the diagnosis is cancer?

One of the basic principles of Parsons' sick role theory is that the ill person is exempt from normal roles and responsibilities and has the right to be cared for by others. As Parsons says: 'Illness is predominantly a withdrawal into a dependent relation, it is asking "to be taken care of"' (1951: 285). This may be relatively unproblematic when applied to adults, but when applied to young people accepting the sick role it may restore the dependent status of childhood, a state from which there is not enough distance to make it acceptable (Brannen et al. 1994). As we have seen, young adults are struggling to establish their independent status, and may not be 'asking to be taken care of'. Indeed, they may instead resist the sick role in an attempt to retain independence. What may, however, happen is that they are forced into a situation where others must take care of them.

Given the nature of many cancers, the duration of the illness and various treatment types, much of this care will of necessity fall on the family of origin as Lynam's (1995) study of young adults with cancer shows. Despite the fact that respondents in her study were older (19–30), she identified the likelihood that the family of origin would be the family of care. She also suggests that the events of this life-stage make the experience of illness qualitatively different from when older adults faced the same diagnosis. As she says:

They had to make decisions about quitting, diminishing, or continuing work or taking leave of absence. The impact of the illness upon the capacity to work, or coping with diminished finances as a result of working reduced hours, became a family event. Some families, usually of origin, because of their own financial or human resources, were more readily able to provide support.

(Lynam 1995: 122)

All the studies cited thus far, whether they apply to ages 15–17 (Brannen, Dodd, Oakley and Storey 1994), 18–24 (Apter 2001) or 19–30 (Lynam 1995) suggest that this life-stage of young adulthood is a transitional period during which family relationships are being renegotiated and independence is being sought. Thus an enforced return to dependent status, made necessary by ill-health, has the potential to throw even the most 'stable' family into chaos. Young adults who have recently claimed their independent status may feel they can only be truly adult away from home as is shown in the following quote from Alec, a young man included in Apter's research:

' You can't really be an adult when you live at home. With your Mom fussing around – well, you're just fighting for space, and can't tell whether you're really independent . . . '

(Apter 2001: 73–4)

In addition, parents will have been used to having had responsibility for their children's health in infancy and childhood. Thus even though a young adult may have become independent and responsible for his or her own health, a tendency to slip back into relationships more appropriate to an earlier life-stage may be difficult to resist.

It would be useful at this point to consider how responsibility for health is negotiated during adolescence. Brannen, Dodd, Oakley and Storey (1994), whose study encompasses the younger end of the age range, say that even at this early stage changes are taking place. They consider the nature of GP and hospital visits during this life-stage and observe that when a parent does accompany a young adult child, it will usually be the mother, and it is more likely that a mother will accompany her daughter than her son. While a mother will see it as appropriate to accompany a daughter to seek medical advice on female health issues, their study suggests that a mother is likely to consider it inappropriate to accompany a son after the age of 16. Waiting outside the consulting room may represent a compromise and allows the young person to consult the doctor in confidence, but the mother will expect a full account after the consultation. Having been involved in health-related decisions and medical consultation throughout their children's lives, mothers in particular may find it difficult to relinquish:

In being excluded from the doctor's consulting room, some mothers fear missing out on important information concerning their children's state of health; either the young people do not ask the doctor the 'right questions' or they do not ask questions at all. Sometimes they fail to pass on any information gained.

(Brannen, Dodd, Oakley and Storey 1994: 97)

Here the situation as it relates to relatively minor illnesses is being addressed. However, when a medical consultation relates to a possible cancer diagnosis, the anxieties can only be more severe. The likelihood is that the young person will still want privacy and will try to assert independence, and that the process of exclusion will be experienced by the parents [mother] as extremely stressful. There is also the question of confidentiality. Given the potential seriousness of a cancer diagnosis young adults may allow their parent[s] to accompany them to a medical consultation, but this will mean that despite being above the age of majority in some cases, they are sharing with their parents medical information which they could choose to keep private.

Judgements may have to be made between 'capacity' and 'majority' during this transition period. Thornes (2001: 15) reflects that while young people over the age of 18, who have the capacity to think independently, have the right to make their own health care decisions, young people between the ages of 16–18 may also have this capacity. According to the Family Law Reform Act 1969, a 16-year-old is considered capable of consenting to treatment without parental consent (HMG 1969). However, if a 16-year-old refused medical treatment, either a parent or the court could override their decision. The situation is further complicated by the Gillick principle (Thornes 2001), which requires clinicians to judge capacity/competence of a young person even under the age of 16 and to then involve them appropriately in decisions.

The sharing of medical information, when the diagnosis is cancer, may result in the need to address sensitive issues not usually discussed openly between young adults and their parents. A cancer diagnosis will frequently have implications for future fertility, thus issues of sexuality and procreation, which usually remain unaddressed between parents and adult children, may have to be confronted. Brannen, Dodd, Oakley and Storey note that while some mothers will help their daughters to obtain contraception, in many families a 'blind' eye' is turned to sexual activity, as the parents may prefer not to be confronted with the knowledge that their son or daughter is sexually active. The right to become sexually active without parental approval, or even knowledge, tends to accompany the independence that comes with joining the workforce and/or leaving home. Yet young adults who are diagnosed with cancer may also find that if independence, normally central to this age group, is lost, then such private activity may become a family concern. Thornes (2001) suggests that parents are often surprised that their adolescent terminally ill child has sexual feelings. If the young person is also separated by the illness from their peers as a source of information about sexual matters this can present a challenge to parents.

The effect on life trajectories

It has been established that young adults are at a transitional and emotionally turbulent life-stage and that families managing any illness diagnosed in young adults will encounter significant additional problems. Given that a diagnosis of cancer amongst any age group carries its own significant psychosocial impact, when these factors are combined the result is likely to produce considerable problems for the family's management of the illness.

Costain Schou and Hewison (1999) consider the drain on 'personal resources' posed by cancer treatment and the impact of this drain on the identity and personal calendars of patients. We have already seen that identity and its construction through a bid for independence are crucial to young adults, and their personal calendars are particularly significant at this life-stage when they should be moving through educational goals, beginning careers and establishing intimate relationships.

The concept of 'identity' is central to our understanding of the impact of a cancer diagnosis at this stage in life. Mishler (1999: 8) argues that the search for an all-encompassing total 'IDENTITY' (original emphasis) is not as useful as the recognition that we are all the sum of a number of 'sub-identities'. While this may become increasingly true during a life where 'identity formation' is the outcome of a series of life events and relationships, at the life-stage which is the focus for this book the default identity, when other identities are lost, may be that of dependent child. Mishler's study of narratives of identity continues by observing that discontinuities and disjunctions in career paths were typical rather than unusual in his research, and he documents 'the centrality of discontinuities in adult identity formation' (1999: 13). However, changing trajectories in adult life may be experienced very differently from changes in young adulthood. As Apter says, 'the term "identity crisis" has largely been associated with adolescence' and she quotes Erikson as arguing that at no other stage of the life cycle are the promise of both finding and the threat of losing oneself so closely allied (2001: 69).

One of the particular issues related to the life-stage of young adults with cancer is that of the tension between their 'life trajectory' and their 'treatment trajectory'. That is, the direction in which they 'should' be heading at this time in their life is threatened by the treatment regime that is forcing them to head in a very different direction. Thus trajectories may be in direct opposition to each other in a way that is thrown into sharp relief by the rapidity of change that would normally occur during this period in a young person's life. Costain Schou and Hewison quote extensively from Rachael, a 41-year-old teacher whose holiday to America was cancelled when her treatment for breast cancer had to be extended. Rachael was clearly disappointed by this, but we may assume that age and experience would afford her the knowledge that there would be another chance to holiday in America after the treatment was over. This case provides an example of a 'discontinuity' as identified by Mishler (1999), who suggests that such disjunctions are to be expected. However, for the young adults whose treatment trajectory conflicts with their life trajectory in terms of education or career, such a setback may seem catastrophic – which indeed it may be in reality; for example, if treatment stops young adults from taking A levels, they may not be offered a place at university. If they are unable to take university exams they may not complete their degree, or if they are unable to attend job interviews they may miss out on career or employment opportunities.

While, with experience, we may realize that opportunities are rarely lost for all time (for example, it is possible to attend university as a mature student), to the young person such setbacks must be unendurable when coupled with concern over illness and recovery and the fact that contemporaries are likely to be moving through those life-stage goals and leaving them behind.

The interruption of the life or career trajectory at this life-stage is also likely to have a profound effect on the young adult's concept of his or her own identity. While older cancer patients are likely to have a well-established identity in their professional or personal life, this is not the case for many young adults. Costain Schou and Hewison consider the primacy of the 'calendar' in Western culture and the importance of 'knowing *who* I am exactly within it' (1999: 83). The centrality of life-plans is what provides a stable source of identity legitimation (Ezzy 1993, in Costain Schou and Hewison 1999). However, the treatment calendar necessitates the formation of new life-plans that clash with the personal calendar of the patient and this can have a profound effect on identity. The cancer diagnosis, according to Costain Schou and Hewison, causes huge disruptions in the life calendars of individuals and it seems likely that this effect is exacerbated when experienced by young adults whose life-plans are likely to be both in crisis and negotiation at this life-stage. The additional effect this has on identity must also be far-reaching, as this will be closely connected to the life-plans which confer identity as a student or in a profession or in an intimate relationship, all of which may be lost through the cancer diagnosis. Thus the loss of such identity-confirming activity will be exaggerated in comparison to those being given a cancer diagnosis at a point in their lives when these identities are more firmly established. As Apter (2001) says, being an adult not only means being able to do 'grown-up' things it also means having a 'grown-up' identity, but serious illness is likely to threaten both. In a table charting the effects of life-threatening illness during young adulthood, Thornes (2001) lists interference with vocational plans and difficulties and discrimination in securing employment. Such effects hinder separation from the family and arguably result in undermining identity.

Acknowledgements

This extract was adapted from Grinyer (2002a: 4–10).

References

Albritton, K. and Bleyer, W.A. (2003) The management of cancer in the older adolescent, *European Journal of Cancer*, 39(18): 2584–99.

Alderson, P. and Morrow, V. (2004) *Ethics, Social Research and Consulting with Young People*. Essex: Barnardos.

Apter, T. (2001) *The Myth of Maturity: What Teenagers Need from Parents to Become Adults*. New York: W.W. Norton and Co Inc.

Arbuckle, J., Cotton, R., Eden, T.O.B., Jones, R. and Leonard, R. (2005) Who should care for young people with cancer?, in T.O.B. Eden, R.D. Barr, A. Bleyer and M. Whiteson (eds) *Cancer and the Adolescent*. Oxford: Blackwell: 231–40.

Arksey, H. (1996) Collecting data through joint interviews, *Social Research Update*, Issue 15, Winter 1996, University of Surrey.

Atkin, K., Rodney, A. and Cheater, F. (2006) Disability, chronic illness, fertility and minority ethnic young people: making sense of identity, diversity and difference, in R. Balen and M. Crawshaw (eds) *Sexuality and Fertility Issues in Ill Health and Disability from Early Adolescence to Adulthood*. London: Jessica Kingsley Publishers: 129–43.

Baldwin, S. (1985) *The Costs of Caring: Families with Disabled Children*. London: Routledge and Kegan Paul.

Balen, A. and Glaser, A. (2006) Health conditions and treatments affecting fertility in childhood and teenage years, in R. Balen and M. Crawshaw (eds) *Sexuality and Fertility Issues in Ill Health and Disability from Early Adolescence to Adulthood*. London: Jessica Kingsley Publishers: 67–84.

Bearison, D. (2006) *When Treatment Fails*. Oxford: Oxford University Press.

Beresford, B. (1995) *Expert Opinions: A National Survey of Parents Caring for a Severely Disabled Child*. Bristol: Policy Press.

Birch, J.M. (2005) Patterns of incidence of cancer in teenagers and young adults: implications for aetiology, in T.O.B. Eden, R.D. Barr, A. Bleyer and M. Whiteson (eds) *Cancer and the Adolescent*. Oxford: Blackwell: 13–31.

Birch, J.M., Alston, R.D., Quinn, M. and Kelsey, A.M. (2003) Incidence of malignant disease by morphological type, in young persons aged 12–24 years in England 1979–1997, *European Journal of Cancer*, 39(18): 2622–31.

Blanchard, J. and Lurie, N. (2004) R-E-S-P-E-C-T: Patient reports of disrespect in the health care setting and its impact on care, *Journal of Family Practice*, 53(9): 721–30.

Bleyer, A., Budd, T. and Montello, (2005) Lack of participation of older adolescents and young adults in clinical trials: impact in the USA, in T.O.B. Eden, R.D.

Barr, A. Bleyer and M. Whiteson (eds) *Cancer and the Adolescent*. Oxford: Blackwell: 32–45.

Brannen, J., Dodd, K., Oakley, A. and Storey, P. (1994) *Young People, Health and Family Life*. Buckingham: Open University Press.

Brindle, D. (2005) Opinion, Society, *Guardian*, 5 January, p. 5.

Costain Schou, K. and Hewison, J. (1999) *Experiencing Cancer*. Buckingham: Open University Press.

Craig, F. (2006) Adolescents and young adults, in A. Goldman, R. Hain and S. Liben (eds) *Oxford Textbook of Palliative Care for Children*. Oxford: Oxford University Press: 108–18.

Crawshaw, M. (2006) The sting in the tail: teenagers coping with sperm banking following a cancer diagnosis, in R. Balen and M. Crawshaw (eds) *Sexuality and Fertility Issues in Ill Health and Disability from Early Adolescence to Adulthood*. London: Jessica Kingsley Publishers: 144–58.

Daly, J. (2006) My friend Kelly was told she had an STI, *Company*, January: 42–3.

Decker, C., Phillips, C.R. and Haase, J.E. (2004) Information needs of young adults with cancer, *Journal of Pediatric Oncology Nursing*, 21(6): 327–34.

Dobson, B. and Middleton, S. (1998) *Paying to Care: The Cost of Childhood Disability*. York: Joseph Rowntree Foundation.

Eden, T. (2006) *Teenagers and Young Adults with Cancer 'The Forgotten Tribe'*, retrieved from: http://www.eolc-observatory.net/information/presentations/flash/teden_280606.swf (accessed 7 July 2006).

Engel. M. (2005) The day the sky fell in, *Guardian Colour Supplement*, 3 December, pp. 18–26.

Enskar, K., Carlsson, M., Golsater, M. and Hamrin, E. (1997) Symptom distress and life situation in adolescents with cancer, *Cancer Nursing*, 20(1): 23–33.

Estelle, C.J. (1990) Contrasting creativity and alienation in adolescent experience, *The Arts in Psychotherapy*, 17: 101–7.

Farrell, C. (2006) Patients' views and experiences of NHS cancer services, National Cancer Service Framework Assessments, Commission for Health Improvement/Audit Commission, retrieved from: http://scholar.google.com/scholar?hl=en&lr=&q=cache:KT_cHj28M4cJ:www.chi.nhs (accessed 8 July 2006).

Fielding, N. (1995) Interviewing, in N. Gilbert (ed.) *Researching Social Life*. London: Sage: 135–53.

Flaherty, M. (2006) *Crossing the Line: Pushing the Limits of Professional Boundaries*, retrieved from: http://www.nurseweek.com/features/98–10/involve.html (accessed 31 May 2006).

Geehan, S. (2003) The benefits and drawbacks of treatment in a specialist Teenage Unit – a patient's perspective, *European Journal of Cancer*, 39(18): 2681–3.

George, R. and Hutton, S. (2003) Palliative care in adolescents, *European Journal of Cancer*, 39(18): 2662–8.

Glaser, B. and Strauss, A. (1967) *The Discovery of Grounded Theory*. Chicago: Aldine.

Grant, J.M. and Roberts, J. (1988) Psychological development: sex and sexuality in adolescence, in T. Harrison (ed.) *Children and Sexuality*. London: Bailliere Tindall: 67–87.

Grinyer, A. (2002a) *Cancer in Young Adults: Through Parents' Eyes*. Buckingham: Open University Press.

Grinyer, A. (2002b) The anonymity of research participants: assumptions, ethics and practicalities, *Social Research Update*, Issue 36, University of Surrey.

Grinyer, A. (2004a) Young adults with cancer: parents' interaction with health care professionals, *The European Journal of Cancer Care*, 13: 88–95.

Grinyer, A. (2005) Personal agendas in emotionally demanding research, *Social Research Update*, Issue 46, University of Surrey.

Grinyer, A. (2006a) Caring for a young adult with cancer: the impact on mothers' health, *Health and Social Care in the Community*, 14(4): 311–18.

Grinyer, A. (2006b) Telling the story of illness and death, *Auto/Biography*, 14: 206–22.

Grinyer, A. In press: The impact of cancer on parents of adolescents and young people, in F. Gibson and D. Kelly (eds) *Cancer Care in Adolescents and Young Adults*. Oxford: Blackwell Science.

Grinyer, A. and Thomas, C. (2001) Young adults with cancer: The effect on parents and families, *International Journal of Palliative Nursing*, 7(4): 162–70.

Grinyer, A. and Thomas, C. (2004) The importance of place of death in young adults with terminal cancer, *Mortality*, 9(2): 114–31.

Grbich, C. (1999) *Qualitative Research in Health*. London: Sage.

Haase, J.E. (2004) The adolescent resilience model as a guide to interventions, *Journal of Pediatric Oncology Nursing*, 21(5): 289–99.

Haase, J.E. and Phillips, C.R. (2004) The adolescent/young adult experience, *Journal of Pediatric Oncology Nursing*, 21(3): 145–9.

Hain, R. (2005) Whose dying is it anyway? Palliative care in adolescence, in T.O.B. Eden, R.D. Barr, A. Bleyer and M. Whiteson (eds) *Cancer and the Adolescent*. Oxford: Blackwell: 203–13.

Hallowell, N., Lawton, J. and Gregory, S. (2005) *Reflections on Research: The Realities of Doing Research in the Social Sciences*. Maidenhead: Open University Press.

Hedstrom, M. and von Essen, L. (2004) Disease and treatment-related distress among children aged 4–7 years: parent and nurse perceptions, in F. Gibson, L. Soanes and B. Sepion (eds) *Perspectives in Paediatric Oncology Nursing*. London: Whurr Publishers: 311–26.

Her Majesty's Government (1969) The Family Law Reform Act 1969, (c.46), section 8.

HERO (Higher Education and Research Opportunities) in the UK: (2005) UK's First Professor of teenage and young adults cancer appointed in Manchester, retrieved from: http://www.hero.ac.uk/media_relations/11209.cfm. (accessed 22 October 2005).

Hinds, P.S., Quargnenti, A.G. and Wentz, T.J. (1992) Measuring symptom distress in adolescents with cancer, *Journal of Paediatric Oncology Nursing*, 9(2): 84–6.

Kline, N.E. (2006) Discussing difficult issues with patients and parents, *Journal of Pediatric Oncology Nursing*, 23(4): 175.

Lacey, H. (2006) A case to answer, *The Independent Extra*, 27 June, pp. 8–9.

Larouche, S.S. and Chin-Peuckert, L. (2006) Changes in body image experienced by young adults with cancer, *Journal of Pediatric Oncology Nursing*, 23(4): 200–9.

Levi, F., Lucchini, F., Negri, E. and La Vecchia, C. (2003) Trends in cancer mortality at age 15 to 24 years in Europe, *European Journal of Cancer*, 39(18): 2611–21.

Lewis, I. (2005) Patterns of care for teenagers and young adults with cancer: is there a single blueprint of care? in T.O.B. Eden, R.D. Barr, A. Bleyer and M. Whiteson (eds) *Cancer and the Adolescent*. Oxford: Blackwell: 241–58.

Lewis, I. and Morgan, S. (2006) Yes or no?: A question of consent, *Contact*, Spring 06, Issue 30: 6–7.

Lynam, J. (1995) Supporting one another: the nature of family work when a young adult has cancer, *Journal of Advanced Nursing*, 22: 116–25.

May, T. (1997) *Social Research: Issues, Methods and Process*. Buckingham: Open University Press.

Michelagnoli, M.P., Pritchard, J. and Phillips, M.B. (2003) Adolescent oncology – a homeland for the 'lost tribe', *European Journal of Cancer*, 39(18): 2571.

Miles, M.B. and Huberman, A.M. (1994) *Qualitative Data Analysis*. London: Sage.

Mishler, E.G. (1999) *Storylines*. London: Harvard University Press.

Morgan, S. and Hubber, D. (2004) Setting up an adolescent service, in F. Gibson, L. Soanes and B. Sepion (eds) *Perspectives in Paediatric Oncology Nursing*. London: Whurr Publishers: 119–40.

National Institute for Health and Clinical Excellence, Guidance on Cancer Services (2005a) *Improving Outcomes in Children and Young People with Cancer, The Manual*. (August 2005). Available on: http://www.nice.org.uk/pdf/csgsp manual.pdf (accessed 20 October 2006).

National Institute for Health and Clinical Excellence, Press release (2005b) *NICE Guidance Set to Improve Services for Children and Young People with Cancer*. Issued: 24 August 2005.

Neville, K.L. (2000) *Mature Beyond their Years: The Impact of Cancer on Adolescent Development*. Pittsburgh, PA: Oncology Nursing Press Inc.

Nishimoto, P.W. (1995) Sex and sexuality in the cancer patient, *Nurse Practitioners. Forum*, 6(4): 221–7.

Parsons, T. (1951) *The Social System*. London: Routledge and Kegan Paul.

Quinn, B. (2003) Sexual health in cancer care, *Nursing Times*, 99(4): 32–4.

Reebals, J.F., Brown, R. and Buckner, E.B. (2006) Nurse practice issues regarding sperm donation in adolescent male cancer patients, *Journal of Pediatric Oncology Nursing*, 23(4): 182–8.

Reres, M. (1980) Stressors on adolescents, *Family Community Medicine*, 2: 32–4.

Ribbens McCarthy, J. (2005) Available on: http://www:jrf.org.uk/knowledge/findings/socialpolicy/0315.asp (accessed 20 October 2006).

Robertson, S. (2006) Lipstick and laughter for teens, *Contact*, Summer 06, Issue 31: 12.

Robson, C. (1995) *Real World Research*. Oxford: Blackwell.

Selby, P., Shah, A., Yates, R. and Leahy, M. (2005) The next 10 years in biomedical science and care for teenagers and young adults with cancer, in T.O.B. Eden, R.D. Barr, A. Bleyer, and M. Whiteson (eds) *Cancer and the Adolescent*. Oxford: Blackwell: 270–82.

Self, M.C. (2005) Surviving with scars: the long term psychosocial consequences of teenage cancer, in T.O.B. Eden, R.D. Barr, A. Bleyer and M. Whiteson (eds) *Cancer and the Adolescent*. Oxford: Blackwell: 183–200.

Shaw, N., Wilford, H. and Sepion, B. (2004) Semen collection in adolescents with cancer, in F. Gibson, L. Soanes and B. Sepion (eds) *Perspectives in Paediatric Oncology Nursing*. London: Whurr Publishers: 141–57.

Smith, L.K., Pope, C. and Botha, J.L. (2005) Patients' help-seeking experiences and delay in cancer presentation: a qualitative synthesis. *The Lancet*, 366: 825–31.

Smith, R. (2004) My last choice, *British Medical Journal*, 329(7460): 1.

Steliarova-Foucher, E., Stiller, C., Kaatsch, P., Berrino, F., Coebergh, J.W., Lacour, B. and Parkin, M. (2004) Geographical patterns and time trends of cancer incidence and survival among children and adolescents in Europe since the 1970s (the ACCIS project): an epidemiological study, *The Lancet*, 364(9451): 2097–3105.

Steyskal, R. (1996) Minimizing the risk of delayed diagnosis of breast cancer, retrieved from: http://www.medscape.com/viewarticle/408807, (accessed 7 July 2006).

Teenage Cancer Trust (2006a) retrieved from: https://www.teenagecancertrust.org/main/healthfacts/ (accessed 20 July 2006).

Teenage Cancer Trust (2006b) retrieved from: https://www.teenagecancertrust.org/main/units/ (accessed 25 July 2006).

Thomas, D.M. (2006) Australia needs to improve management of young people with cancer, Press release, retrieved from: http://www.ivyrose.co.uk/Health/show_di.php?id=1027 (accessed 28 April 2006).

Thomas, D.M., Seymour, J.F., O'Brien, T., Sawyer, S.M. and Ashley, D.M. (2006) Adolescent and young adult cancer: a revolution in evolution? *Internal Medicine Journal*, 36(5): 302–7.

Thornes, R. (2001) *Palliative Care for Young People Aged 13–24 Years*. London: National Council for Hospice and Specialist Palliative Care Services.

University of Manchester (2006) Sperm banking gives teenage cancer patients hope for the future, retrieved from: http://www.manchester.ac.uk/aboutus/news/pressreleases/sperm, (accessed 9 March 2006).

Ussher, J., Kirsten, L., Butow, P. and Sandoval, M. (2006) What do cancer support groups provide which other supportive relationships do not? The experience of peer support groups for people with cancer, *Social Science and Medicine*, 62: 2565–76.

Viner, R. (2003) Bridging the gaps: transition of young people with cancer, *European Journal of Cancer*, 39(18): 2684–87.

Wallace, W.H.B. and Brougham, M.F.H. (2005) Subfertility in adolescents with cancer: who is at risk and what can be done? in T.O.B. Eden, R.D. Barr, A. Bleyer and M. Whiteson (eds) *Cancer and the Adolescent*. Oxford: Blackwell: 133–54.

West Midlands Paediatric Macmillan Team, (2005) *Palliative Care for the Child with Malignant Disease*. London: Quay Books.

Whelan, J. (2005) Support for teenagers grows, *Contact*, Winter 05, Issue 29, p.12.

Whiteson, M. (2005) A right not a privilege, in T.O.B. Eden, R.D. Barr, A. Bleyer and M. Whiteson (eds) *Cancer and the Adolescent*. Oxford: Blackwell: 1–10.

Woodgate, R.L. (2006) The importance of being there: perspectives of social support by adolescents with cancer, *Journal of Pediatric Oncology Nursing*, 23(3): 122–34.

Woman's Hour (2006) Interview with Dr Guy Makin, Manchester University, 9 March, retrieved from: http://www.bbc.co.uk/radio4/womanshour/01/2006_10_thu.shtml, (accessed 9 March 2006).

Zebrack, B. (2006) Young adult cancer survivors: shaken up, getting back, moving on, in R. Balen and M. Crawshaw (eds) *Sexuality and Fertility Issues in Ill Health and Disability from Early Adolescence to Adulthood*. London: Jessica Kingsley Publishers: 221–33.

Index

RETHINKING EXPERIENCES OF CHILDHOOD CANCER
A Multidisciplinary Approach to Chronic Childhood Illness

Mary Dixon-Woods, Bridget Young and David Henney

This book offers a radical critique of existing psychosocial research on children's experiences of cancer and proposes an alternative view informed by recent interpretive perspectives. Exploring topics from obtaining a diagnosis of childhood cancer through to sharing decision-making and communication, it reviews a wide-ranging body of research and theory on childhood, chronic illness, and cancer. The book also examines research that has focused on how parents and other family members experience childhood illness.

Written by a sociologist, a psychologist and a practising paediatric oncologist, this book is unique in its approach and provides key reading across traditional disciplinary boundaries. In particular, the book highlights the emerging contribution of interpretive work to understanding chronic childhood illness and further develops the dialogue that has only recently emerged between the sociology of illness and the sociology of childhood.

Rethinking Experiences of Childhood Cancer is key reading for researchers, students and practitioners in the fields of social science, childhood studies, nursing, medicine, mental health care, social work, clinical psychology and other professions allied to medicine, and will also be of interest to families who have been affected by childhood cancer.

Contents: *Approaches to childhood and childhood cancer - Obtaining a diagnosis of childhood cancer - Having childhood cancer - Late effects of childhood cancer - Families' experiences of childhood cancer - Communication in childhood cancer - Shared decision making in childhood cancer - Conclusions - Bibliography - Index.*

244pp
ISBN-13: 978 0 335 21255 2 (ISBN-10: 0 335 21255 7) Paperback
ISBN-13: 978 0 335 21256 9 (ISBN-10: 0 335 21256 5) Hardback

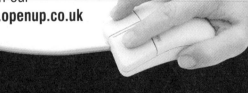